In Defense of Human Dignity

LOYOLA TOPICS IN POLITICAL PHILOSOPHY

Thomas S. Engeman
Series Editor

This series originates in the Frank M. Covey, Jr., Lectures in Political Analysis. The Covey Lectures are delivered annually at Loyola University Chicago and published in a series by the University of Notre Dame Press. Frank Covey, a distinguished lawyer and Loyola alumnus, endowed the lectures to promote the study of political philosophy, in the expectation that this enquiry would contribute to human understanding and political justice. The books in the Loyola Topics in Political Philosophy series offer a number of responses of prominent scholars to issues addressed in the Covey Lectures. Each volume contains an introductory essay by the Covey lecturer and a concluding reflection on new issues raised by the contributors. The intention of the series is to offer the best current scholarship to teachers and students, as well as to general readers.

IN
DEFENSE
OF
HUMAN DIGNITY

Essays for Our Times

ROBERT P. KRAYNAK
GLENN TINDER

editors

UNIVERSITY OF NOTRE DAME PRESS

Notre Dame, Indiana

The editors and the publisher are grateful to John Rawls for
permission to include his essay "A Well-Ordered Society."

Library of Congress Cataloging-in-Publication Data

In defense of human dignity : essays for our times / Robert P.
Kraynak and Glenn Tinder, editors.
p. cm. — (Loyola topics in political philosophy)
Includes bibliographical references and index.
ISBN 0-268-03170-3 (cloth : alk. paper)
ISBN 0-268-03164-9 (pbk. : alk. paper)
1. Philosophical anthropology. 2. Dignity. 3. Man (Christian
theology) 4. Dignity—Religious aspects—Christianity.
I. Kraynak, Robert P., 1949– . II. Tinder, Glenn E. III. Series.
BD450.I48   2003
128—dc21
2002013299

CONTENTS

INTRODUCTION

Defending Human Dignity: The Challenge of Our Times   1
Robert P. Kraynak

CHAPTER ONE

Against Fate: An Essay on Personal Dignity   11
Glenn Tinder

CHAPTER TWO

Kant on Human Dignity   53
Susan M. Shell

CHAPTER THREE

"Made in the Image of God":   81
The Christian View of Human Dignity and Political Order
Robert P. Kraynak

CHAPTER FOUR

Between Sanctity and Depravity: Human Dignity   119
in Protestant Perspective
John Witte, Jr.

CHAPTER FIVE

A House Divided, Again: Sanctity vs. Dignity   139
in the Induced Death Debates
Timothy P. Jackson

CHAPTER SIX

Are Freedom and Dignity Enough?   165
A Reflection on Liberal Abbreviations
David Walsh

CHAPTER SEVEN

A Well-Ordered Society   193
    John Rawls

CHAPTER EIGHT

Saving Modernity from Itself: John Paul II on   207
Human Dignity, "the Whole Truth about Man,"
and the Modern Quest for Freedom
    Kenneth L. Grasso

AFTERWORD

Facets of Personal Dignity   237
    Glenn Tinder

Contributors   247
Index   249

In Defense of Human Dignity

Defending Human Dignity: The Challenge of Our Times

ROBERT P. KRAYNAK

The defense of human dignity has been a perennial theme of philosophers and theologians, but it takes on new and special urgency in our own times. Over the course of the last several centuries, much of the world has embraced an ideal of civilization that measures its progress by claims of improving the human condition and enhancing human dignity. The results, as everyone knows, have been astonishing. In the political arena, the great revolutions waged in the name of human rights have raised the status of millions of people by giving them new opportunities for individual freedom and democratic self-government. In the intellectual and cultural spheres, the scientific Enlightenment has given mankind new powers to unlock the secrets of the natural universe and helped to make us, in the words of Descartes, the masters and owners of nature. As workers and consumers in a modern economy, we have seen the industrial revolution, combined with modern technology, unleash the productive energies of countless working people and raise their standard of living to unprecedented levels. All of these achievements have given individuals and nations a heightened sense of their dignity by making them aware of their basic human rights and giving them the power to control their destiny and to master their fate.

While enhancing human dignity in these respects, modern civilization has also engendered doubts about the overall improvement of humanity—doubts that have multiplied in the last century as the modern project has unfolded. In the areas mentioned above—politics, science, technology, and industrial development—as well as in other areas, the advances of modern civilization have created new problems, including new threats to human dignity. In trying to describe these threats, social critics sometimes speak of living in a "dehumanized" world where individuals no longer count and the collective forces of the modern world diminish our humanity. Though cries of "dehumanization" can sound melodramatic and self-pitying at times, the term points to genuine threats to human dignity that come from many sources—from the all-powerful centralized state, from new technologies, from an impersonal society in which we are disconnected from our fellow citizens, from a disenchanted world of soulless materialism, from a loss of contact with the natural environment, and from the fear of being "lost in the cosmos" where man seems all alone in an indifferent universe. These examples remind us of broad trends operating in the modern world that explain why a growing number of observers—including the authors of this volume—think that the major challenge of our times is to recover a true and authentic understanding of human dignity and to defend it against threats from modern civilization. Before turning to the defense, however, let us consider some of the threats in greater detail.

The political problems arise from the two most powerful forms of government in the modern world: totalitarianism and liberal democracy. Though by no means morally equivalent (as radical critics of Western democracy sometimes claim), the two systems have a common source in the trends of modern mass society. Unlike older political structures—such as the governments of ancient city-states, feudal kingships, or the great multiethnic empires of the past—modern nation states are mass phenomena. They rest on a social base of the broad mass of people who are no longer tied by ancient roots and traditions to a particular locality, to an ethnic group or tribe, and to a social class that gave them a sense of their place in the world. Instead, modern mass societies rest on aggregates of rootless and traditionless individuals, all claiming to be unique and special, but who are, in reality, just like their anonymous neighbors in their mundane pursuits. Such individuals have greater opportunities for personal achievement and social mobility than previous generations, but they lack strong horizons and clear identities, leaving them with few moral resources to resist the pressures of mass conformity and few associations to resist the power of the centralized state that arises to serve and to control them.

In extreme instances, modern mass society leads to totalitarianism, which is made possible not only by crises, such as war and economic depression, but also by the breakdown of local institutions and secondary associations, which leaves the isolated individual standing frightened and alone before the total state and its tyrannical rulers. In more mundane fashion, mass society produces the vast welfare state bureaucracy of modern democracies, which has also been described as a type of despotism but of a kinder and gentler type than totalitarian dictatorship. In the words of Alexis de Tocqueville, the centralized bureaucratic state can become a "soft despotism" that imposes a stifling regime of equality, uniformity, and guaranteed material security on people, debasing them without quite allowing them to admit it by weakening their wills with degraded dependency and discouraging their initiative. Compounding the problem are the seductive materialism and hedonism of modern capitalism, which act like a gigantic feeding machine for mass tastes and popular culture. In the world created by the welfare state and the consumer-entertainment society, few people have time or energy left for responsible citizenship and difficult duties, not to mention the more refined aspirations of high culture. These trends, unleashed by modern mass society and exploited by the modern state and modern industry, are threats to human dignity because they subvert the character of human beings as rational and responsible agents and as virtuous and free citizens.

If we turn to science and technology, we can see other threats to human dignity that have attracted widespread publicity. Everyone is familiar with the cloning of animals and other techniques of genetic engineering, and the scientific and business communities are now speculating about the potential uses of the human genome project. These developments raise direct and immediate questions about the central issues of human dignity: Does the human species have a distinct and privileged place in the cosmos that conveys special duties and rights on human beings? Does each one of us have a unique destiny and moral worth that needs to be protected against perverted science? Such questions also underlie the great debates about life and death in medical ethics—debates about abortion, euthanasia, fetal tissue research, and the manipulation of genes and cells to prevent diseases and possibly to arrest the aging process or to abolish death itself. In wrestling with the moral aspects of modern technology and medicine, we need to raise the discussion to the highest possible level by recognizing that what is at stake is not merely human health and longevity or new technical skills and commercial enterprises but the dignity of man as a distinct species in the natural universe and the moral and spiritual worth of individuals within the human species.

Ironically, some of the most disturbing movements growing out of the modern scientific revolution and modern philosophy recognize very clearly what is at stake. I am referring to certain brands of radical environmentalism and to the practical ethics movement of Peter Singer. They welcome the opportunity to convince the public that the status of human beings should be lowered in relation to other animals or other forms of organic life. One of their prime objectives is to treat the whole concern with human dignity—with the superior dignity of human beings and with the intrinsic worth and sanctity of human individuals—as an irrational prejudice, the prejudice of "species-ism," which unduly privileges human beings in the natural universe. Many radical environmentalists view mankind as a kind of blight on the planet, the great violator of the otherwise benevolent order of nature, who deserves to be humbled by shock tactics of various sorts. They trace the arrogance of species-ism not only to the Cartesian project of making men the masters and owners of nature but also to the biblical claim that man is made in the image of God and placed at the peak of creation with a grant of dominion over the earth and to the claim of Greek philosophy that humans are at the top of nature's hierarchy because they have rational souls. Though one may wonder if any environmentalist really believes that all species are equal—that, for example, saving a pet rabbit is just as important as saving a human child—one must take seriously the theoretical and practical challenges to human dignity posed by radical environmentalism. Even the more moderate and rational brands raise important questions about our proper place in the natural order that deserve thoughtful responses.

Following the same line of thought, the practical ethics movement associated with Peter Singer requires an adequate response by philosophers and theologians. Singer is notorious for minimizing the difference between animals and humans and claiming that higher types of animals with sentience—including "the much maligned chicken"—are worthy of more respect than humans with deficient brains or other handicaps. He has even advanced the shocking proposal that every newborn human child should be given a one-month probation or trial period during which time the parents may decide to keep or to destroy the child if they do not find the child up to snuff. It seems ironic that someone like Singer, who has raised consciousness about the suffering of animals to new heights, has also given greater respectability to infanticide. But, if modern society has no clear understanding of what constitutes human dignity, why should Peter Singer be condemned for drawing the logical conclusion and defending the proposition that some human beings are *not* worthy of life and liberty? Singer's utilitarian ethics and subversion of traditional hierarchies are in a way predictable outgrowths of the threats to human dignity in much of modern thinking.[1]

If one pushes a bit further, one may wonder if modern science and modern philosophy as a whole have enhanced or undermined the dignity of man. On this topic, some of the most penetrating insights were offered at the end of the nineteenth century by Friedrich Nietzsche, who observed that the theories of Copernicus and Darwin have greatly reduced the stature of man by displacing him from the center and peak of the universe and by encouraging us to belittle ourselves:

> Has the self-belittlement of man ... not progressed irresistibly since Copernicus? Alas, the faith in the dignity and uniqueness of man, in his irreplaceability in the great chain of being, is a thing of the past—he has become an *animal*, literally and without reservation or qualification, he who was, according to his old faith, almost God (a "child of God," [or] "God-man"). Since Copernicus, man seems to have got himself on an inclined plane—now he is slipping faster and faster away from the center into—what? into nothingness? ... *All* science (and by no means only astronomy ... of which Kant made the noteworthy confession: "it destroys my importance") ... has at present the object of dissuading man from his former respect for himself, as if this had been nothing but a piece of bizarre conceit.[2]

Nietzsche's point is that modern science displaced the medieval Christian worldview, which formerly gave human beings a lofty status in the universe, both physically and morally. He also notes that some modern philosophers such as Immanuel Kant have tried deliberately to save human dignity through a transcendental philosophy of freedom. Nietzsche's insight about the downward slide of man in the modern age may come as a surprise to those who think of Nietzsche as a cynic, for it shows how deeply he cared about the dignity of man. It also forces us to think about everything in modern life that degrades or debases the human spirit and to ask if the defense of human dignity is "a thing of the past," as Nietzsche says with considerable regret. Is the concern with enhancing the dignity of man something that people used to worry about, but we no longer worry about because the effort seems futile or unnecessary? Could anyone in the twentieth century write an essay like Pico della Mirandola did five hundred years ago when he published his "Oration on the Dignity of Man" and expect to receive a favorable hearing? Or is human dignity something we care about but take for granted as a cultural inheritance that no longer needs defending?

It is precisely to restore the question of human dignity to the central importance it once occupied that this volume was conceived and developed. In a sense, the project began twenty years ago when Glenn Tinder delivered the Covey Lectures at Loyola University of Chicago and chose as his topic the threats to personal dignity in modern times. Tinder's original lectures were published as a book entitled *Against Fate: An Essay on Personal Dignity*. That work has been presented here in an edited version and may be considered the launching pad and motivating force behind this volume.

According to Tinder, the "dignity of the individual" is "the quality by virtue of which every person is to be treated as an end and never merely as a means"; he identifies this principle as "the primary intuition of Western moral consciousness and indispensable to liberal democracy." Tinder traces it to Christianity and to Kantian ethics and defends it in his writings because he feels that this primary moral intuition is in danger of being lost. By analyzing the threats that the external forces of "fate" pose to the unique "destiny" of every person, Tinder hopes to re-instill reverence for the transcendent dignity of the individual. He also points the way to a brand of politics that avoids the modern illusions of mastery and accepts the God-given limits of human existence.

The six essays that follow Tinder's piece develop his themes as well as offer alternative perspectives on human dignity and its political and ethical implications. In a brilliant essay, "Kant on Human Dignity," Susan M. Shell discusses one of the crucial philosophical underpinnings of Tinder's moral idealism. She shows how much Kant is responsible for shaping the way the modern Western world thinks about human dignity. With sympathy and critical insight, she argues that Kant conceived of "dignity" as the inherent worth of every human being instead of the rank of a person in a hierarchy or a chain of command—a novel proposition that enabled Kant to link human dignity with democracy and individual rights.

In my own essay, "'Made in the Image of God': The Christian View of Human Dignity and Political Order," I take a different approach by focusing on the way that the Bible and the great Christian theologians conceive of human dignity. I argue that the foundation of human dignity in the Bible is the *Imago Dei*—the divine image in man—and that its meaning has evolved over the centuries from a hierarchical to a democratic conception. While noting the reasons for this change, I also point out the problems for modern Christians as they try to balance the affirmation of everyone's infinite worth with the demands for spiritual and moral perfection.

John Witte, Jr., sheds further light on the Christian conception of human dignity in his essay, "Between Sanctity and Depravity: Human Dignity in Protestant Perspective." He highlights Martin Luther's claim that man has a dual nature—*simul justus et peccator,* both righteous and sinful—and explains how this conception has contributed to the rise of modern democracy. Despite his basic optimism about the harmony of Protestantism and democracy, he offers sober advice to those who would defend human dignity and human rights without taking into account the fallen nature of man.

Timothy P. Jackson brings the debate about human dignity up-to-date in a provocative discussion of human life issues in medical ethics. He refers to our present society as "A House Divided, Again"—comparing our predicament to Abraham Lincoln's—because several prominent proponents of abortion and euthanasia, such as Peter Singer and Ronald Dworkin, have put the concept of "dignity" (understood as personal autonomy) over against the "sanctity" of life (understood as the inherent worth of persons who need to love and be loved by others). Following the example of Abraham Lincoln, Jackson seeks to give us theoretical and practical guidance in the present moral confusion.

Like other contributors, David Walsh is concerned with the assumptions about human dignity that underlie contemporary liberal democracy. In reflecting on the meaning of "liberal abbreviations," he uses his subtle moral sense to show how the liberal democracies of the West continue to live off the moral capital originally established by Christianity and its notion of the transcendent dignity of the person. Walsh warns that modern liberals are increasingly unwilling to admit this fact, putting their future in jeopardy unless they renew those resources and make the proper, spiritual defense of human dignity their primary concern.

As a counterpoint to Walsh's appeal to the spiritual sources of human dignity, we have republished a classic essay by John Rawls on the moral basis of "a well-ordered society." For Rawls, the moral basis is "a Kantian conception of equality," which gives "equal respect and consideration" to every human being as a moral person capable of acting on principles of justice and of developing a unique life plan. From this premise, Rawls goes on to develop his influential and widely debated vision of a just society that permits inequalities only insofar as they benefit the least advantaged members of society.

In dialectical fashion, we move back to the spiritual dimension of the human person by one of the greatest champions of human dignity in our times, Pope John Paul II. Assessing the pope's contribution, Kenneth L. Grasso argues that "the dignity of the human person" is the central theme of John Paul's pontificate, from his Christology to his social teachings to his pastoral work. In presenting the pope's brand of Christian personalism, Grasso shows how many elements of Christian theology and moral philosophy have been blended together by John Paul into a new and coherent synthesis that gives us "the whole truth about man" and enables us to weigh the benefits and dangers of modern freedom.

Taken together, these essays are designed to stimulate thought about the critical issues of human dignity raised in Glenn Tinder's original essay. They force us to ask questions that have been forgotten or taken for granted. What exactly do we mean by human dignity and related notions such as human "sanctity" or "worth"? What trait or attribute gives us our special character as a species: Is it the possession of reason, free will, an immortal soul, capacities for love and justice, the ability to suffer pain, a special relation with God? Is dignity something we share with other animals that are also capable of feeling pain and sensations? How is human dignity justified: Is it essentially a philosophical, religious, or cosmological claim? What implications does one's conception of human dignity have for ethics and politics? Are there limits and dangers in the contemporary appeals to human dignity? All of these questions are discussed on various levels by the authors of this volume, and the variety of religious and philosophical perspectives should give the reader some sense of the power and complexity of the issue. Above all, they should remind us that the concern with the dignity of man is not "a thing of the past," as many fear, but a living issue of primary importance to all of mankind as well as to citizens of modern democratic society.

Notes

1. See Peter Singer, *Rethinking Life and Death: The Collapse of Our Traditional Ethics* (New York: St. Martin's Press, 1995), and *Practical Ethics* (Cambridge: Cambridge University Press, 1993).
2. Friedrich Nietzsche, *On the Genealogy of Morals,* part 3, sect. 25, pp. 155–56, trans. Walter Kaufmann and R. J. Hollingdale (New York: Vintage, 1967).

CHAPTER ONE

Against Fate:
An Essay on Personal Dignity

GLENN TINDER

Prologue: The Dignity of the Individual

My main concern in the following pages is with what is now usually called "the dignity of the individual," or, in the terminology of Immanuel Kant, with the quality by virtue of which every person should be treated as an end and never merely as a means. This I believe to be the primary intuition of Western moral consciousness and indispensable to liberal democracy. My concern with this concept stems from my conviction that it is not only important but is being lost. It is a deeply mysterious idea. It affirms the dignity of *every* individual. But how can it be said that someone who is ruined in body, mind, or character—as many individuals are—bears an inviolable dignity? The idea is necessarily in tension, moreover, with political, economic, and administrative practice, which involves strong pressures to treat every individual simply as a calculable and expendable resource. It is not surprising that personal dignity has been terribly and extensively violated in times as troubled as ours and that it seems often to be little more than a cliché of popular rhetoric.

"Fate" I use as a term to designate the great world forces that lay waste to individual lives and tell us that an individual is merely a plaything of war, economic dislocation, tyrannical power, disease, and the myriad chances that defy all personal and political precautions. Fate is the impersonal and the antipersonal, coming in varied forms but always seeming to bear an unchallengeable message: that a single person is negligible in power and value alike. In words made commonplace by familiarity, fate is "meaningless" or "absurd." It may be fragmented and come upon us in disjointed circumstances, or it may be massive and unified, even predictable. It may be experienced in recurrent jolts or in a holocaust that devours us. It is always alien and dangerous.

To withstand fate, we must find ways of reaffirming personal dignity. I employ the term "destiny" to this end. In common usage, destiny is often equated with fate. Occasionally, however, the term is used to suggest that destiny, even if preordained and severe, is somehow congruent with humanity in a way that fate is not. It is sometimes suggested, for example, that we may fail to fulfill our destinies. This would not be said of fate. Moreover, destiny is never meaningless or absurd. Your destiny is the life you were meant to live. It is a story that makes sense. To the extent that world events take the form destiny, one is lifted up, rather than crushed, by the powers and forces of history. In short, destiny enables a person to stand forth from surrounding circumstances as an end, not merely a means.

The contrasting concepts of fate and destiny should help to illuminate the present historical situation. If these concepts work as intended, they will enable us to see how personal dignity is threatened in the modern world and how it may be defended. To deal in a short essay with matters so vast and enigmatic may sound presumptuous. Let me say, then, that I do not try in a fundamental way to be original. I try merely to make in a new way certain points that are very old.

These old points are Christian. My views of personal dignity and of history are Christian, although my arguments appeal to natural reason and natural intuition, not to faith. Indeed, I would have little confidence in the ideas I set forth if they were drawn merely from my own mind rather than from Christian traditions. What is original lies in the concepts employed. I have cast the Christian view of humanity and history in terms that are new and might thus be persuasive for those not attracted by Christian terms. In this way I hope to make it possible for a vision that is profound and ancient, but unacceptable to many in our day, to cast light on our times.

At the core of my argument is the idea that fate is ironic: although it seems to come upon us from without, we ourselves are the main authors of our fate. Swept up in a drive to master the natural and social worlds, and ignoring the finitude and imperfection of man, we encounter human limits suddenly and disastrously. Fate is made up largely of the unexpected consequences of our own actions. The drive to mastery underlies modern phenomena like technology, revolution, and the prevalence of ideologies. As a consequence, nature, society, and history all have taken on fated qualities. Looking on nature as nothing more than material to serve human convenience and avarice, for example, we have lost the sense, expressed in both Hebraic scripture and Greek philosophy, of the deep harmony of humanity and nature; results are evident in the noxious and unsightly environment so often created by modern industry. Striving forcibly and swiftly to reshape society according to such perfectly valid ideals as liberty and equality, we find ourselves in an era of bureaucracy and totalitarianism. In our determination to direct the course of history we have lost the sense of continuity necessary for seeing the human past as a single story. All of this is ironic, but not accidental. It originates in our pride—a pride seen not among radicals alone but also, in various forms, among liberals and conservatives.

The fatefulness of our times is deeply hostile to personal dignity. This hostility is sometimes violent and frightening, as in the widespread use of political torture. But it is sometimes subtle and beguiling. Thus industrialism has provided a fate that, for many in Western Europe and America, is enjoyable. It has bestowed on vast numbers of people comforts and distractions that kings could not enjoy a few centuries ago. But these are fateful pleasures. They divert us from the tasks of selfhood with more cunning and charm, but not with less effect, than the wars, revolutions, economic breakdowns, and other disasters that punctuated the twentieth century. In all of its forms, however, fate challenges us to reaffirm and defend personal dignity. To this end we must understand personal dignity, and I shall try to show how this can be done through the concept of destiny.

Here again, however, we encounter an obstruction caused by our will to mastery. Destiny, like fate, is ironic and is not made according to human will and desire. The irony of destiny is that even though it is the life of the intimate and sacred self, it is given to us, not as a natural necessity, but as a personal possibility and moral demand. Dignity consists in the possession of a destiny and is affirmed through fidelity to individual destiny.

Our situation is thus that in our technological and revolutionary pride we have lost our sense of destiny and have fallen under the dominion of fate. Yet there are possibilities of renewal. Fate is something we have made, not simply suffered, and destiny continues to be demanded of us. The possibilities of renewal, moreover, are not just for individuals but for all of us together. Although destiny is personal, it is also universally human and becomes accessible only as we recognize our responsibility for the common life of humanity, a life that links generations in history. We need today, in place of the crumbling idea of progress, a reawakened consciousness of the proper form of the life of humanity in time, our common destiny. To be open to and to act upon the demands of universal destiny is "the true political art," a phrase Plato applied to Socrates' conduct of his own life and the subject with which the essay concludes.

Fate

The Irony of Fate

A symptom of our situation today is the appeal of the unassuming phrase, "human scale." The powers and organizations that govern us, the realities that make up our world, are too vast. Every person is overshadowed by corporations and governmental bureaucracies, powers and superpowers, and human multitudes unimaginable in numbers and cultural diversity. We cannot experience these things as we do trees or houses or anything else with definite and perceptible proportions. We can hardly even conceive of them, although we know well enough that they are real. Anyone undeluded by power or pleasure feels small, in fact negligible, in size, power, perhaps even in worth. It is not only the bulk of these monstrous realities that disturbs us; it is also their apparent autonomy. They are seemingly out of control. Our future is not our own. Yet to say that the great powers of the world are out of control does not mean merely that they are out of your control and mine. We sense that they are not controlled by anyone. We are told occasionally that some kind of elite—business executives, perhaps, or bureaucrats— rules us. Society is depicted in the lurid colors of conspiracy. Although analyses of this kind often purport to be alarming, they are in fact strangely consoling. They make the world seem relatively human and comprehensible.

Such consolation is illusory. Elites today probably attain no purposes more distant and sweeping than the expansion of their own wealth and prestige. It is even questionable whether the tyrannies closely identified with one name, like Stalin or Hitler, are altogether controlled by the man bearing the name. The Soviet Union long survived the death of Stalin, and Hitler owed his power largely to his skill in reflecting German fears and passions.

Elitist theories do, however, contain a glimmering of truth. Fate is largely a human product. The vast events and powers that overshadow our lives have been created by humanity itself. Wars, economic dislocations, bureaucracies, and tyrannies all are human products. That they are produced by humans striving to impose their will on events is the irony of fate. Although fate is something that befalls us, it is also something that we ourselves have brought into being. It is not surprising, of course, that people should bring harm on themselves. What is surprising is that they should persistently experience this harm as having struck them from without.

Fate is brutal factuality, and our world is fated because it is dominated by powers that are wantonly inconsiderate of the core of our humanity, the distinct personality. How uncanny, then, that these brutal facts are human. Again and again it is said that the world today, or some worldly phenomenon, is inhuman. It is true that much in our world is inhuman in its indifference to personal well-being and integrity. But in its origins, its structure, and its energies it is pervasively and manifestly human. Never before has the world been so human. The environment for most of us is almost completely a human artifact or a conglomeration of human artifacts; enclaves of nature survive only with determined protection. The most fateful events of our time have not been earthquakes and storms but revolutions and wars, movements that sweep over the earth like plagues but are purely, if devastatingly, human.

An irony, however, is not simply a juxtaposition of discordant circumstances. In the words of Reinhold Niebuhr, an irony consists of "apparently fortuitous incongruities in life which are discovered, upon closer examination, to be not merely fortuitous."[1] Historical events and conditions are ironic, then, if there is a hidden link between them. What is the link between the human source and the inhuman quality of our situation today? It is, I suggest, an exaggerated conception of our own power and goodness.

Fate and Pride

Pride calls forth fate by clouding our understanding of the world around us. Failing to perceive our own limitations, we fail also to perceive the mystery and independence of the realities we seek to control. In this way pride leads, in its blindness, to actions that entail unforeseen consequences. These are experienced as fate. The greater our pride and the more ambitious our programs of action, the more massive the fate from which we are likely to suffer.

Although human beings are naturally inclined to be proud, the illusion that we can understand all reality and organize and dispose of it as we please has been greatly encouraged by science and industry. So spectacular have been our technological successes that we have come to see ourselves as masters, potentially if not actually, of all nature and history. This self-confidence was affirmed in the doctrine of progress and, a handful of dissident thinkers aside, was for a century or two virtually universal. During this time the fate we are now experiencing was blindly created. Even today, tenacious in our illusions, we tell ourselves that we have a right to "choose our own destiny." What have the industrialists, revolutionaries, and other proud creators of our world failed to see or to take sufficiently seriously? Some rather elementary, but significant, conditions.

For one, our immanence—or, to use a more commonplace word, our "immersion"—in reality. We cannot rise above the universe and survey it altogether. We must investigate things like explorers traveling through virgin territory on a raft. We cannot see even the course of the stream we are navigating, much less the entire territory we are exploring. This is to speak of our finitude and of the impediments it places on action. Just as we cannot see all of reality in a glance, neither can we anticipate all the consequences of our acts. Pride might be defined as illusory transcendence. Neglecting our immanence, it acts blindly. In this way, it exposes us to fate. The state of things in Russia at the end of the twentieth century perfectly illustrates the point. The economic and political chaos prevailing in that tormented country was not created by an earthquake or plague but by a group of supremely self-confident Russians.

To disregard human immanence is to blind oneself not only to the dangers of incautious action but also to the mystery and plenitude of being. Only what we call "objects" are fully comprehensible and controllable, and pride therefore objectifies. Pride typically strives to understand the spiritual as material, the individual as general, the spontaneous as necessary. Pride in its major Western forms is intolerant of all that cannot be rationally explained and deliberately organized. It was not because the French bourgeoisie in the early years of the twentieth century were philistines that they were outraged by painters such as Cézanne and Renoir; it was rather, we may surmise, because they sensed that such painters were uncovering aspects of reality, such as shimmering light, that did not lend themselves to rational comprehension and control.

If human beings are reluctant to acknowledge that they are finite, they are even more reluctant to admit that they are morally flawed. Proudly, they do not notice, or they somehow explain away, the selfishness, callousness, and cruelty that abound wherever they congregate. They banish "sin" from the vocabulary of literate discourse. Then, oblivious of the evil in their own nature, they trust in their power. In this way they become vulnerable not merely to miscalculation but to their own malicious impulses. Such proud innocence can be so undiluted that its results are viewed as purely accidental. Thus the Bolsheviks of 1917 naively assumed not merely that human ignorance, but that human iniquity as well, were passing historical phenomena. Thus they took little care to provide against these phenomena, for example, with checks and balances in the political order they created. As a result, not merely did they fall short of their goals; they produced a singularly terrible regime. But how was Stalin's government regarded by most of those who laid the groundwork for it and then became its victims? Not as something they had in their blindness willed but as a monstrous misfortune.

Pride, in sum, is willful blindness to human immanence, to the mystery of being, and to sin. It is a striving toward an ascendancy in which human beings possess the wisdom and righteousness of gods and have all reality at their disposal. It is perhaps the strongest of all human inclinations. Frequently, however, it is restrained or concealed. We could

not inhabit the earth together unless the will to ascendancy were in various ways curbed by the necessities of common life. Pride thus may live
underground, as it were, concealed by social courtesies and nourished
by small and inconspicuous victories. Or it may become collective, as in
bellicose patriotism, racial bigotry, and ideological intransigence.

Further, pride at times gives way altogether. When this happens,
the end sought becomes, in place of inordinate expansion of the self,
the virtual eradication of the self. People become inclined to give up,
not merely power and domination, but all responsibility. The motive is
physical and spiritual security—guaranteed by someone else. Those
governed by Dostoevsky's Grand Inquisitor (an exemplar of pride)
desired "bread, miracles, and authority." They desired a world without
risks, solitude, or doubt, and this entailed the idolatry implicit in absolute obedience. The underlying moral state, replacing pride, may be
called "self-abandonment."

Self-abandonment arises from despair. Losing all self-confidence,
one seeks to be relieved of one's very selfhood. Despair assumes many
forms. It is enacted in sensuality, dissipation, and suicide; it is present
in the obsessive busyness in which there is no thought, happiness, or
hope; and it creates the silent subservience and unreasoning belligerence that upholds tyrants.

Self-abandonment is probably as common as pride, although it is
apt to arise only as pride is defeated. It does not, however, lessen the
reach of pride or limit the reign of fate. For one thing, it is probably
never pure, unmixed with any form of personal or collective pride. But
even at its purest, self-abandonment in some only makes room for pride
in others. People flee into the arms of fate. Some mistake fate for a
stable, comprehensible, and agreeable world, while others see it as it is
but welcome the destruction it promises. In 1933 some Germans followed Hitler because he held out prospects of power, wealth, and status;
others did so in a desperate effort to evade political and spiritual responsibilities they felt incapable of meeting. In 1945 many remained loyal
to Hitler in the face of national defeat and that must have been in some
cases because he showed the way to a fiery and mindless death.

The hidden link between the humanity and inhumanity of fate,
then, is the inclination of every person to be something other than a
mere human being: to gain the autonomy and transcendence of a god
or the irresponsibility and insentience of a thing. To be merely human

is to live by bread, which no social arrangements can assure absolutely; by faith and intellect, with all of the uncertainties attendant on both; and in a state of freedom, thus bearing responsibility for the character of one's life. It is not surprising that we recoil from circumstances so uncomfortable. In doing so, however, we call forth the insubordinate events and powers that constitute fate.

It is understandable that fated situations often give rise, simultaneously, to feelings of guilt and of helplessness. This paradoxical state of mind is described with great power by Dostoevsky in *Crime and Punishment*. Raskolnikov knew that he was fully responsible for murdering the old pawnbroker and her sister. He could not blame his crime on his poverty or the squalid circumstances in which he lived. Yet he was driven to the crime by a force so compelling that it was "as though someone had taken his hand and pulled him along irresistibly, blindly, with supernatural strength."[2] A broadly similar paradox was experienced in America during the war in Vietnam. Multitudes of Americans felt that the actions their government were carrying out in Vietnam amounted to a crime of immense proportions. Equally widespread, however, was the sensation of being caught in a vast misfortune, a fate of which Americans, no less than the Vietnamese whose homes and lives they were destroying, were the victims. "So bewildered were Americans *by what was happening to them and by what they themselves were doing,*" as one writer remarked, "that many came to believe that both in Indo-China and at home the United States had been overtaken by a wholly accidental and therefore wholly absurd fate."[3]

Pride, Suffering, and Hope

The nature and the fateful consequences of pride, as well as the strength of pride in our time, may be further clarified by reflecting on contemporary attitudes toward suffering. People today are fiercely intolerant of suffering. This is indicated by how intimate and open the relationship between suffering and resentment has become. Those who suffer typically assume that someone else is responsible for their suffering—even when they themselves clearly bear some responsibility, as in the case of lifelong smokers who sue tobacco companies on account of the illnesses they have contracted. To suffer is in a certain sense to be humbled; people in complete command of their lives would not suffer. Our intolerance of suffering, then, reflects our pride. And it brings to our attention another aspect of the irony of fate, that in proudly repudiating suffering, modern humans have contributed to the vast amount of suffering experienced in our fated times.

Of course suffering can never be completely acceptable. If it were, it would not be suffering. But it has often been regarded—as by ancient Hebrews, remembering their decades in the wilderness, ancient Greeks, taught by the tragedians, and Christians, centered on the Crucifixion— as bearable and potentially fruitful. Such patience has largely passed. In capitalist advertising and leftist rhetoric alike, suffering is denied all legitimacy. Life should be enjoyable; insofar as it is not, remedial steps should be taken without delay. Capitalists think of these steps in terms of economic productivity and individual acquisition, social reformers in terms of institutional reform. From both sides any indifference to a life physically secure and enjoyable is regarded as anomalous and retrograde. The idea that suffering ought to be patiently, even hopefully, borne (Paul said, "We rejoice in our sufferings")[4] is incomprehensible to both "conservatives" and "liberals," to both private entrepreneurs and governmental administrators.

How have our views on this matter come to be so uniform? Leaving aside the fact that lessening, or at least promising to lessen, suffering is economically and politically profitable, several reasons are discernible. Each of these tells us something about modern pride.

First, our power of avoiding and postponing suffering is far greater than ever before in history, and this has intensified our pride. We are less respectful of the inevitable than were past ages; we are less cognizant of the limits on our power. We do not merely strive to lessen suffering, however. One cannot miss in modern rhetoric the alluring thought of a world from which suffering has been altogether banished. Such a world would not only offer a life that is reliably enjoyable; it would testify to human mastery. The indefinite continuance of suffering strikes us as humiliating; it casts doubt on our understanding and command of the realities around us.

Not only have science and technology made suffering seem unnecessary; our rationalistic self-assurance has made it seem meaningless. Suffering has often been seen as a mystery in which is hidden the meaning of life. For the authors of Jewish scripture, the forty years of wandering in the wilderness were not an exercise in futility or a sign of their failure to manage their lives efficiently; the wandering testified to their ultimate destiny and mirrored the will of a merciful God. To acknowledge a mystery, however, requires humility. For most people today, the world around us has only the meanings we assign it and impose upon it. Adverse circumstances contain no mystery, and we may pit ourselves against them without compunction.

Finally, not only do we see ourselves as sovereign in power and the universe as potentially a mirror of our purposes, but we also are confident of our moral innocence. We do not deserve to suffer. For traditional Christianity, as expressed in the myth of original sin, every person was guilty in the very orientation of his being, an orientation away from God and toward the self and the world. Hence, apart from the suffering of Christ, there was no innocent suffering. For many intelligent and responsible people today, most suffering is innocent. Misdeeds are committed, to be sure, but these are exceptional and owing to remediable mental and social derangements. The prospect of human cosmic sovereignty thus causes us few misgivings.

It is true that considerable disillusionment occurred in the twentieth century. Our self-confidence has been shaken not only by the war, tyranny, and economic chaos marking the earlier part of the century, but also by the global turmoil and the domestic crime and social disintegration experienced in almost every nation at the century's close. So much the more remarkable, then, is the manifest fact that the most literate groups in the West remain, by and large, children of the Enlightenment. They are disappointed and perplexed but trustful still of human power. They look around them, not for meanings which rule and overrule our calculated actions, but for ways in which our command of events can be restored.

Thus throughout our political, economic, and social lives, the judgment implied constantly and in countless variations is that human suffering is avoidable, meaningless, and undeserved. Twentieth-century Americans have seen innumerable examples of the trivial and destructive ends for which men purposely or thoughtlessly use their technological and industrial power. Most of us seem still to believe that the happiness of the human race waits mainly on our identifying and solving the main problems that plague us. In this regard, the differences among the ideologies are surprisingly slight. Supporters of free markets, of careful measures of social reform, and of radical economic and

political reconstruction are at one in seeing suffering as an object of conquest. To scarcely anyone, at least among those whose profession is
speaking and writing, is it a source of wisdom or a redeeming mystery.

With all of our self-confidence, however, our hope is by no means
boundless. Not only does despair lurk at the edges of our life, given the
history of our times. We avoid despair only through self-assurance, and
that is not quite the same as hope. Self-assurance is the feeling that
everything is under control, or can be, at least. All problems are soluble.
Hope, on the other hand, is confidence that all will finally be well,
although not necessarily due to human foresight and action, or in fulfillment of our conscious desires, or even in a way that is empirically
manifest in personal lives or historical events. Summarily, assurance
rests on the belief that the universe is rationally comprehensible, hope
on the faith that the universe in its depths is mysteriously in accord with
humanity in its depths.

The weakness of modern hope helps to explain how it is that our
age is proud and yet strangely close to despair. When our self-assurance
is challenged, nothing remains. In the face of fate, our inner balance is
precarious. In our time, peoples have sought self-assurance through reli-
able political, social, and economic systems—in socialism, for example,
or else in free markets—and, as their desperation increased, they have
resorted to awesome historical agents, such as great nations, parties,
and leaders.

The themes of suffering and hope are unfolded in the drama of
Doctor Zhivago. Pasternak recounts, in essence, the resistance of one
man to the fate set in motion by the Russian Revolution of 1917, a resistance dependent on a willingness to suffer. Zhivago thought in the first
stages of the Revolution that the way might be opened for the human
possibilities so harshly denied by the czarist regime. The revolutionaries, however, soon displayed an implacable historical willfulness and,
along with this, an absence of hope, of openness to destiny. The Revolution turned into a fate which laid waste the Russian land and people
and Zhivago's own life as well—his medical practice, his personal relations, his health. Little survived for Zhivago but a capacity for hope—
a hope painfully severed from the Revolution and deprived of all
reasonable prospects but retained as an indefeasible spirit of invulner-
ability to worldly mischances and grief.

In his political detachment, Zhivago was a strange and suspicious figure (like Pasternak himself) in the eyes of the Communist rulers. In his isolation he was weak and exposed. But fate did not have the last word, even though it disrupted the order of his existence and finally destroyed his life. Immersed in suffering, his own and that of people he loved, he lived without despair his own singular life.

It is tempting, mixing fiction and reality, to contrast Zhivago and Lenin: on one side vulnerability, on the other absolute power; on one side hope, on the other self-assurance; on one side receptivity, on the other will; finally, on one side a personal life carried on, with all of its suffering, in what Pasternak refers to as "the air of freedom and unconcern that he [Zhivago] had always emanated,"[5] on the other side, judging from Lenin's final and futile efforts to block the rise of Stalin and the Party bureaucracy, defeat by fate.

People all over the world have found political inspiration in Lenin. Scarcely anyone thinks of Dr. Zhivago as representing a serious political stance. Soviet rulers showed by their hostility to Pasternak, however, that they knew better. They knew that Zhivago embodied an ethos deeply at odds with the political principles they represented, principles which in their magnification of human will were only an extreme version of the political faith of modern man.

Destiny

Selfhood as Destiny

Destiny is selfhood—authentic and enduring (qualities conveyed by the word "soul")—as a temporal unfoldment. So far as I live a destiny, all that I do and suffer has a place in a life experience that is a gradual disclosure of personal identity. Within the scope of a destiny, nothing merely befalls me, nothing is merely outward and accidental. Every occurrence plays a part in the actualization of my essential being. Augustine's *Confessions* dramatizes the destiny of an African churchman living in the fateful final days of the Roman Empire, and many novels, like *Crime and Punishment* and *Doctor Zhivago*, tell us a great deal about the destinies lived by modern people.

No one, of course, lives a life manifest as pure destiny. No one can discern in every accident of life the drama of self-actualization, and death usually seems to come too soon or too late. The world surrounding us often is, or appears to be, brutally indifferent to the fragile identities individuals try to establish. In a few individuals, such as religious martyrs or patriotic heroes, even torture and death apparently enter into the substance of an exalted selfhood. But most lives, as far as we can tell by objective observation, are repeatedly deranged by assaults of fate.

The concept of destiny implies that selfhood is not merely an abstract and immutable identity transcending the struggle to embody that identity in a concrete life. It is also the struggle itself, for a full human being incorporates all of his past, all that has gone into his making. Hence it must be said, not that one *has* a destiny, but that one *is* a destiny.

The limits of reason in the face of destiny are apparent. A man or woman is not something that can be definitively known and simply is what it is, like a tree or a house. A destiny is not a quality, like a color or shape, that belongs to such an object. A person is always more than anyone can know about him. A person is not only one who is in some measure known but also the one who knows, and as the one who knows also the one who inquires and discovers—a "thought-adventurer," as D. H. Lawrence said. A man or woman is even more than this, however, for your identity is in some measure a matter of choice. You can censure some of your qualities and can change. To conceive of a *being* who is essentially *becoming* is difficult. But to think of a concrete person, a being who is a destiny, this is what must be done.

While destiny is never fully apparent, it is real in every life and is known in some degree to all of us. Just as no one has lived a life free altogether of fate, so no one has lived a life lacking all traces of destiny. You may wonder, for example, whether you have chosen the right vocation. Granted, this may be thought of merely as a life activity bringing personal pleasure, plentiful remuneration, and the satisfaction of serving others. But the term "vocation" suggests more than this: it is a call or summons. To think seriously of your vocation, or of the vocation of someone you greatly care for, is to be aware that a person's life is not to be used in any way that is pleasant or profitable or even in any way that happens to be helpful to others. It is subject to more ultimate demands. The sense of destiny is particularly poignant in the consciousness of having missed one's vocation. This is not merely regret at not being happier or more useful. It is awareness of not having lived the life one was given to live.

Common feelings for friends, mates, and offspring also exemplify our familiarity with destiny. The feeling that a close and enduring marriage does not originate in mere human preferences and choices is apt to be tritely expressed yet is a compelling intuition. Some relationships cannot be thought of as though they might never have been. And one's children often evoke a sense of destiny. It is easy to feel that the world is a far worse place for them to inhabit than you had anticipated, or that they have not become the sort of people you wanted them to become. But it is difficult, even impossible, to regard them as nothing more than products of a biological accident or an imprudent decision.

Good novels sometimes make us conscious of destiny. When they do, it is by brushing away the details that in actual life do not clearly cohere as either fate or destiny and that thus obscure the meaning of our deeds and sufferings. Not that novels always show us destiny fulfilled. They may show us destiny forsaken: Nicholas Stavrogin, for example, in contrast with Pierre Bezhukov. But either way, they dissipate the fog of senseless circumstance and hint of meanings that the life of a person has or ought to have. The satisfaction given us, that of feeling that it had to be so, comes from sensing more strongly than we ordinarily can the necessity inherent in destiny and in the fate that signifies a destiny neglected or defied.

Any kind of storytelling can be a way of searching for the meaning that constitutes a destiny. The opaque facts of daily life are sorted out and rearranged in an effort to discover their personal significance, which is to say, how they reflect a fate willed unintentionally, if proudly, or a destiny accepted and lived. There are also less wise and gentle ways that human beings have of trying to understand or effect the subordination of circumstances to personality. Astrology is one of these.

Interest in astrology is apt to be widespread in times of spiritual turmoil, and it mirrors an awareness both of fate and of destiny. The former is more obvious: for astrologers, everything from the movement of the stars to the details of daily life is fixed in the patterns of an impersonal universe. But followers of astrology are not simply devotees of doom. If the patterns of the universe can be descried before they have had their way, they can be made to serve the ends of personal life. Such an inference is illogical, but spontaneous and nearly inevitable. And it can evoke an image of destiny—of the universe, apparently overwhelming in its infinitude and indifference, actually in subordination to human selfhood.

Do we not, moreover, sometimes see in political violence an effort to convert fate into destiny—an effort that is activist and directed toward history rather than the physical universe? An assassin, for example, may be not only poor and powerless but obsessed with his own insignificance. People of wealth and fame represent an alien and menacing world. The act of assassination presents a prospect of shattering these fateful surroundings. For a few days in 1963, a world that occasionally seemed to be contained in the destiny of John F. Kennedy appeared suddenly to have been violently rearranged according to the destiny of Lee Harvey Oswald. And how many revolutions have been lifted up and carried forward on a wave of faith in some version of historical destiny?

That destiny is authentic selfhood helps explain why the connotations of necessity and freedom are both paradoxically present in the concept of destiny. The connotation of necessity is so pronounced that destiny is often confused with fate, and the words are used interchangeably. But the necessity inherent in fate is experienced as external and coercive, while the necessity in destiny is personal. What is destined is what must occur if you are to be yourself. "Here I stand, I can do no other." Luther's apocryphal words point dramatically to the personal character of the necessity inherent in destiny. Considering merely what outward circumstances allow, rarely has Luther or anyone else been confined to a single choice. But considering who you are and must be, every alternative may melt away. What is at stake is not a personality structure that one might alter or vacate as though it were a house. Selfhood is not something that is used; it is an end rather than a means, and it is an end of the kind that cannot be set aside in favor of other ends. It is the only end that matters. "For what is a man profited, if he gain the whole world and lose his own soul?"

Living one's destiny, then, is an unconditional moral imperative. Nevertheless, it cannot be done simply by adhering to moral rules. You must live your own particular and distinctive life. Moral rules only alert you to the kind of imperatives that in every case must arise from your own unique situation. Someone who in every thought and act perfectly satisfied the moral law but did nothing more than that, would be a phantom of rectitude, lacking the mystery and plenitude of humanity. But generality is not the only limitation inherent in the moral law; imperfect applicability is another. This is true especially in politics, where complex circumstances often make it impossible to follow all the relevant rules. Even if the moral law were perfectly applicable to every concrete situation, obeying it in detail would be beyond anyone's power. Human beings are incapable of perfect righteousness; this is the gist of Paul's critique of Jewish reliance on the Torah. Until we die, all of us must stand in some degree condemned before the majesty of the law.

A destiny may be accomplished, however, in spite of such failures. This is the theme of the Christian doctrine of forgiveness and an insight not wholly foreign to the Hellenic mind, as shown by the Oedipus drama. The moral transfiguration that Paul envisioned is only in part a matter of visible conduct; in part it is accomplished in the mystery of the Resurrection. "It is no longer I who live," as Paul said, "but Christ who lives in me."[6] The moral law bespeaks our subjection to an absolute claim. This claim can be fulfilled, however, only as a destiny—a destiny incorporating both failures and forgiveness.

Destiny is freedom, and its intrinsic necessity is in part the inviolable demand of freedom upon us: that you embrace your identity as deliberately and lucidly as you can. But freedom is not caprice. It is living your own life rather than the life prescribed by another, under the authority of your own authentic being and not at the dictate of casual impulses or prospective pleasures. Hence destiny entails living at once freely and as you must.

The concept of destiny pertains to persons and not to objects in space and time. Accordingly, it cannot be pointed to or precisely described, as can natural phenomena. It must be spoken of evocatively, equivocally, symbolically. Hints of destiny are contained in the classical triad of values—goodness, truth, and beauty. If I seriously contemplate the idea goodness, for example, I will almost certainly begin to sense that the person I actually am is not the same as the person I ought to be and that I should concentrate upon reaching that unrealized and beckoning identity. Truth also provides such an intimation. It does this by telling us that truth is worthy of unconditional respect; whether it is useful or pleasant is irrelevant. How could such respect be appropriate unless ultimate being were congruous with the striving of the self

toward its own authentic reality, toward its destiny? Beauty offers sen-
suous suggestions of this congruity. A painting by Matisse, for example,
shows us a world that seems perfectly proportioned to the tastes and
temper of the essential self, and a Beethoven symphony seems to delineate the pure and unchecked movement of a destiny.

The idea of life is often invoked in an effort to characterize human
existence in its fullness. But destiny is not life, at least not life alone. We
recognize this in our scorn for those who would sacrifice anything
simply to stay alive. We recognize it also in our respect, not only for
martyrs and military heroes, but even for those who risk their lives for
an insignificant end, such as reaching the top of a particular mountain.
We have an intuition that a person can lose life itself yet somehow gain
substantial being. Indeed, if destiny did not somehow transcend and
encompass death there could be no destiny, since everyone must die.

Destiny is paradoxical. It may take the form of righteousness
achieved in spite of guilt (affirmed by Paul as a possibility inherent in
the mercy of God), truth found in ignorance (suggested by Socrates'
serene professions of ignorance in confrontation with death), beauty
apparent in ugliness (as in the face of Abraham Lincoln), dignity inseparable from horror and suffering (encountered in heroes of tragic
drama such as Oedipus). In the presence of a destiny we feel that all is
as it ought to be, although we may be unable to explain in what way or
why this is so.

Destiny does not belong exclusively to great figures, however. We
have an inkling that it belongs to every human being without exception. We say that each one possesses "infinite value" and is "an end and
not merely a means." We speak of "the dignity of the individual." What
do we mean? Not that every person in his present, manifest being com-
pels respect, for that is not so. Nor do we mean that every person commands respect by virtue of his potentialities, for we affirm the dignity
of those who are mentally retarded and hopelessly ill. We cannot be
referring to any objective reality or natural potentiality, to anything that
can be pointed to or precisely described. Teleology is an inadequate
metaphysic of destiny because it is necessarily inegalitarian, as in Aristotle, and cannot explain the dignity of those, such as the severely
retarded, whose potentialities (at least in the usual sense of the term)
are relatively slight.

Although a destiny is thoroughly personal—my destiny, or yours—
we should not infer that it is mine and in no way yours, or yours and
in no way mine, as though destiny were divisive. A destiny is antithetical
to fate but not to another destiny. Indeed, Christian theology suggests
that in some sense all destinies are one. In Adam's sin there occurred
the fall, not of Adam alone, but of every person. And in Christ's suffering the penalty owing for every misdeed in human history was in some
sense paid. The Resurrection spelled enduring life not just for Christ
but for every human being willing to enter into the common humanity
that Christ represented. How this could be is rationally inexplicable.
Yet we have an intuition of its truth in the experience of love: my own
being is not curtailed but rather is established and enlarged through
relations with those I love. Through love, the individuality and the unity
of persons mysteriously coalesce. And there are no clear limits to the
range of this principle. Love should be universal, in some way embracing all human beings; such, at least, is a familiar principle. It is only
slightly recasting this principle to suggest that I may, as I begin to make
out the contours of my own story, feel that I am seeing dimly the contours of the story of all humanity.

The Irony of Destiny

To speak of choosing your own destiny, as we so often do, reflects a misunderstanding of human beings and their powers—a misunderstanding at the heart of the present crisis of civilization. Perhaps people can
create styles of life and control the general order of their daily existence.
But their destinies must be given them. This is indicated by the word
"destiny" itself, with its connotation of necessity. One carries out a destiny under constraint and not as a matter of play, improvisation, or spontaneous self-expression. The constraint comes from the life one feels
called upon to live. That destiny is required of one, rather than freely
chosen, is evident when fidelity to a destiny requires risking one's life.
This happens frequently, as with young people in a nation at war or citizens confronting a tyrant, and when it does happen the selfhood
implicit in a certain course of conduct may become a sovereign that can
command any sacrifice. People do not invent so inexorable a master.
The givenness of destiny is also disclosed in the ways we think of

personal identity. Even in this self-assertive age people speak of dis-
covering, not creating, themselves. They are concerned with a selfhood
that is not yet fully real and yet in some sense is established and
ordained, since the task is to find it. This paradox, which defines the
structure of destiny, is embodied in the commonplace phrase "finding
yourself" and is stated more dramatically in the maxim that you must
become who you are.

We should be careful, however, not to sever the concepts of destiny
and freedom. Even though our destiny is required of us, living that destiny is freedom. It is not in arbitrary choice, but in the act of creation,
that we realize freedom. That act occurs when someone brings forth a
reality (perhaps a work of art or perhaps merely thoughtful performance of an ordinary daily task) that asserts its singular being apart from
every other such being and in doing so defines and discloses the distinctive being of the creator. In that act one is exalted by the consciousness of stepping forth from dark scenes of struggle and indecision
into light and reality. To be free is to be yourself, and to be yourself is
to be creative. Freedom and creativity in the last analysis are identical.
Creativity, however, is an object of hope and not of will. It depends on
insight ("inspiration") of a kind that cannot be deliberately called forth.
To contemplate the greatest creative figures, and of their having lived
as though under the orders of a transcendental authority, we realize that
freedom is given, as destiny is given, and contains nothing that is willful or capricious. And we perceive that freedom, creativity, and destiny
are ultimately the same.

Matching the irony of fate, then, is the irony of destiny. Fate comes
upon us from without, and it comes destructively, as a violent or seductive enemy of personal being. Yet fate is willed by the person and the
peoples who suffer it. Destiny, on the other hand, is selfhood, the temporal unfoldment and free enactment of one's authentic being. Yet
unlike fate, destiny is given (or withheld, from those unready to receive
it) and cannot be willed.

By what or whom is destiny given? Not by nature, however we conceive of nature: if as a system of universals, the singularity of destiny
would be inexplicable; if as a causal order, the necessity inherent in destiny would be indistinguishable from that of fate; if as a vital force,
destiny would be reduced to mere life. Destiny does not consist in the
fulfillment of potentialities, for a person's potentialities are not, as we

may imagine, a complete and harmonious version of that person latent in nature. They are indeterminate (we read back into someone the potentialities for doing what has already been done), far too manifold and discordant all to be realized, and many of them destructive. Destiny reveals humanity as genuinely temporal and this means, as Henri Bergson brought out so eloquently in his great *Creative Evolution,* going beyond all prior rational determinations both in fact and in norm.

Nor is destiny given by society. If it were, real conflict between the individual (that is, destiny) and society would be impossible. It can be argued that this indeed is the case, that every apparent conflict between individual and society is really a conflict within society. Thus, Socrates was only acting out the disintegration of Hellenic culture, Jesus the humanization and universalization of Judaism. Such an argument would not be wholly wrong. But it would ignore the same reality that is left out of account if destiny is interpreted as a product of nature: the single, irreducible, and distinctive personality. When I take on the responsibility of living my own singular destiny I know that the very responsibility sets me apart from society and requires me to look critically upon the beliefs society offers me and the acts it asks of me. And when I contemplate my destiny I know that it has a mystery and plenitude which make it more than the set of forms and forces I call "society."

Destiny is given by something beyond nature and society, something we may call "transcendence." This is a term with religious overtones, and these are appropriate to the concept of destiny. If we are not mere natural or social accidents, for whom the good is only what we like, the true only what is useful in the way of belief, and the beautiful only a delightful fantasy, then we have our origin in transcendence. Attitudes partaking of awe and trust are inseparable from the realization of this condition. Transcendence can be given the name of God, and Paul expressed a powerful sense of destiny, reflective of a Christian faith in divine providence, when he said that *all things work together for good to them that love God.*[7]

Destiny need not be given any particular creedal definition, however. As a Christian, I believe that the relationship between humanity and transcendence is fully and truly disclosed in Christ. At the same time, I do not believe that Christians alone have access to transcendence. All, in diverse ways, may touch the hem of Christ's garment. Christ as Logos is present in all beautiful art, true thought, and righteous action. Destiny is a call on every person, and wide ranges of human experience tell us that adherents of various creeds are able to answer that call. Did not Plato, Alexander the Great, Buddha, and Muhammad have destinies?

Indeed, it is manifest in the history of literature and philosophy that the call of destiny can be answered even by adherents of no specific creed. "Transcendence" is a word with agnostic (but not atheistic) connotations. Reduced to its most slender proportions, the term enables us to acknowledge the mystery of our origins without involving ourselves in doctrinal or ecclesiastical commitments. Some might question whether a whole life can be lived, or even a whole philosophy formulated, without any such commitments. Socrates' life, however, to mention only one instance, seems to demonstrate the possibility, however exceptional its realization may be. In any case, the term "transcendence" performs a crucial negative function: it warns us against tracing our identities back to any finite source, such as a nation, a party, or a leader, which would be idolatrous and degrading. That the danger is not merely theoretical is shown by the worshipful regard in which nations (such as Nazi Germany), races (the so-called Aryan race, for example), intellectual leaders (like Marx), and political heroes (Lenin, Mao Tse-tung, and Che Guevara) have been held in recent decades. One who lived a destiny agnostically would not lack a consciousness of something sacred undergirding and illuminating existence. This consciousness, without being expressed in any creedal or liturgical forms, would be inherent in the person's sense of the authority of destiny.

In restraining the impulse to worship human agencies, the concept of transcendence guards the sense of unconditionality that is present in an awareness of destiny. In striving to discover my own identity, I am not interested merely in who I *happen* to be, in a self that is no more than a product of circumstances. Such a self would be accidental. I seek acquaintance with my essential being, the content of the inviolable necessity that belongs to destiny. I must look beyond all circumstances, whether natural or social. All of this can and must be said as well of my search for the essential being of someone I love: I do not love a mere accident of natural evolution or social development. The concept of transcendence stands in the way of the crime human beings have committed in countless forms throughout history—the crime underlying all crime—that of reducing the essential human being to an accidental manifestation: to the slave, the barbarian, the heretic, the worker, the capitalist, the Jew, the black.

In sum, the concept of transcendence puts us in an altered relationship with reality. The new relationship may be called "receptivity."

Transcendence and Receptivity

In the age of exploration, science, industry, and revolution—the age that has brought us to our present fateful impasse—the human stance has been more often one of command than of receptivity. People have aspired to ascendancy, whether through intellectual research, economic enterprise, political action, or some combination of these. They have looked on the natural and human realities about them as nothing more than materials lying at hand, available for investigation and use. They have looked on their own psyches in the same way—as comprehensible and controllable, hence at their own disposal. As a result, transcendence has been tacitly or openly denied.

Despite numerous disappointments, these attitudes continue to reign in our minds, prompting reliance on human determination and reason and inducing an insensitivity to destiny. Many are discouraged, but not to the extent of radically questioning the modern project of subordinating all reality to human will. Even most self-styled conservatives go no further than arguing that we must be more cautious if we are to command events effectively. Humility is understood as little more than circumspection. The idea of an altered relationship with being itself has entered the minds of some philosophers and theologians (Karl Jaspers, Martin Buber, and Karl Barth, for example) but has not shaped the imagination of any major ideological group.

I suggest that the central practical issue of modern life is whether in our struggle to extricate ourselves from fate we only intensify our drive toward universal mastery. The corresponding intellectual issue is whether we persist in regarding reality as entirely objective, as made up exclusively of things we can know and control. The issue may be clarified by examining two major forms of receptivity, humanistic and religious.

Humanistic receptivity is a readiness for destiny that does not rely on doctrines concerning transcendence or on forms of worship. It is availability for the life one is called upon to live but it claims no knowledge of the source of that life. It is thus agnostic, although reverent and open. Given a clear understanding that the difference between the two kinds of receptivity is one of degree, it can be said that humanistic receptivity has not congealed as faith and is therefore relatively anthropocentric.

The supreme exemplar of humanistic receptivity is Socrates, moving toward death without terror or anguish, yet ignorant (according to his own professions) of ultimate realities and indefeasibly rational and inquiring. Socrates' receptivity is manifest in his unremitting availability, in the conduct of his philosophic and civic life alike, to the claims upon him of the ultimate good. It is manifest also in the dialogical relationships that he sustained with human beings even at the cost of his life.

A systematic philosophy that is particularly congenial to humanistic receptivity was worked out, over two thousand years later, by Immanuel Kant. According to Kant, we cannot demonstrably know either that God does or does not exist, hence both religious dogmatism and atheism are out of place. Presupposing a strict definition of knowledge, we are bound to be agnostic. Nonetheless, ultimate being is not beyond all insight and surmise. It enters human awareness in various ways— in the consciousness of duty and in the experience of sublimity, for example. Although ultimate being cannot be scientifically known, it governs our lives by drawing us toward truth and holiness. Humans should be uncompromisingly rational, holding free of all dogma, religious and atheistic alike. They should at the same time live in an exploratory and hopeful relationship with ultimate being, or transcendence. Humanistic receptivity is at once transcendental and skeptical. Using Kantian foundation stones, the German philosopher Karl Jaspers worked out a systematic philosophy of humanistic receptivity.

Religious receptivity entails a more definite commitment and hence involves certain concepts of transcendence, that is, theological doctrines. Such concepts often come into conflict with receptivity. It is not clear that this happens necessarily, however. Even so uncompromising a believer as Saint Augustine declared that we believe in order to understand. In other words, faith calls forth rational inquiry. Hence, just as believers must acknowledge the possibility of reverent doubt, as with Socrates, so humanists must acknowledge the possibility of receptive faith.

In the Christian view, all that makes up fate—not only alien and destructive historical forces but even death—has come from the efforts of human beings to create their own destiny rather than live the destiny given them. Mythically described in terms of Adam's eating of the fruit of the tree of the knowledge of good and evil, in contravention of a divine ban, they try to take their lives away from God and into their own hands. In consequence, deprived of the life given them by God, they find their lives under the shadow of a final horror, that of death.

The life of Jesus, for Christians, was pure destiny. Jesus was the Messiah in that through his life all human beings were given access to their own destinies. His crucifixion and resurrection delineate the basic pattern of every human destiny: life gained through death and joy through suffering. Not that the life of Jesus was untouched by *appearances* of fate. In the Crucifixion, he seemingly suffered so fearful a fate that his followers thought his mission had been obliterated. For the first Christians, however, this impression was suddenly and unexpectedly dispelled. The Resurrection became a symbol of the faith that through the Crucifixion God had established his presence at the heart of fate, thus making it possible for each one to enter into the darkness of fate without being destroyed.

This faith is expressed by construing the life of Jesus as the axis of history. All earthly events lead to and follow from that single sovereign event. This is not mere pious exaggeration, lacking all logic. A life that is pure destiny cannot be within history; history must be within that life. And if that life is God's and is open to humankind, then it affects every person. It redirects history and transforms the human situation. Henceforth, the life of Jesus is not merely a dramatic memory, like the lives of Julius Caesar, Leonardo da Vinci, and other great, but purely human, figures. It lays out the possibilities and imperatives facing every human being. Jesus brought a transfigured universe—"new heavens and a new earth."

The difference between humanistic and religious receptivity, then, concerns the source of destiny. Socrates' superiority to fate derived from his certainty of something he could not name or describe. Christian martyrs such as Paul the Apostle and Thomas Becket found in Christ the certainty that enabled them to walk unharmed in the furnace of fate. This difference can be usefully discussed but not rationally resolved.

Those on the two sides can clarify the alternatives before them through inquiring communication but cannot show by logically compelling arguments that one position or the other should be adopted by everyone. It is destiny, so to speak, that decides. We should be wary, however, of assuming that the humanistic version of transcendence, by avoiding the infinite complexities of theology and liturgy, offers a simpler and easier way of living our destinies than does the religious version. It may be that it offers a peculiarly straitened and arduous way, and that few are given the power and imagination to follow it successfully.

Man against Nature and Humanity

Industrialism and the Failure of Receptivity

It is a major premise of modern culture that human afflictions are due primarily to nature, not to human wrongdoing. The task before us is therefore that of subduing nature. This premise sustains our confidence in human will and power. It absolves human beings of responsibility for the tragedies of history and makes it possible to believe that with the growth of science, technology, and industry life will become far better, finally perhaps even paradisiacal. It also makes it possible to believe that the extension of human power need not be over human beings. Nature will be governed by a spontaneously cooperative human race.

Marxism is illustrative. The meaning of history is held to lie in the conquest of nature. Conflict among humans is not caused primarily by defects in their own character. The hatreds of class for class and nation for nation derive, first of all, from the scarcities that inevitably set people against one another; they derive also from the necessity, if these scarcities are to be overcome, for the kind of ruthless mass mobilization that capitalism, in fulfillment of its historical function, carries out. Once nature has been brought under control and material plenty realized, the human situation will be transformed. It will be possible, indeed necessary, for human beings to work and live cooperatively. Class conflict will melt away and with it national rivalries and coercive government.

Marxism is only an insurrectionary, and particularly powerful, version of the modern political faith. Most Americans and Europeans have for a long time assumed that advancing industrialism will eventually bring happiness and social harmony. While a few have come to question the advantages of continuous and unlimited technological and industrial development, they are dissenters from a common faith. The controversies between left and right, between intellectuals and business executives, may cause us to forget how much binds them together. Although the two sides often differ as to the best way of organizing industrial power and the ends to which it should be devoted, seldom do they differ concerning the beneficence of industrial power itself. Both assume that industrial and human progress are broadly coincident. Marxism has appealed to many because of its intellectual force and its rebellious cast. In a certain way, however, it has played a harmonizing role. It has expressed the distaste many have felt for the business ethos and capitalist culture while allowing them to accept unreservedly the basic assumptions of industrial civilization.

Enthrallment with industrial progress is understandable, for it is difficult not to think that technology and industry mark a necessary stage in human destiny. Nature threatens humanity in more ways than one, and it is worse than idle to dream of a life of pastoral peace, innocent of technology and free of industrial imperatives. Nonetheless, the value of technological and industrial development depends on what it is governed by—whether by will or destiny.

The goal set by will is the conquest of nature. To undertake that conquest, however, is to misconceive at the same time nature and human power. To speak simply, nature is not an object of comprehension and control. We cannot, as Kant shows, reach a beginning point in time, an outermost boundary in space, or an indivisible particle of matter, all of which we would have to do in order to declare that all is known. But if our knowledge is essentially incomplete, then our actions are necessarily taken in partial ignorance. We cannot, even in principle, foresee all of their consequences. Hence the unpleasant surprises attending the progress of technology and industry: not only physical phenomena such as foul air and pervasive poisons, but social phenomena like alienation, family disintegration, and a meretricious and shallow culture. These are not accidents of a sort we will finally eliminate. Insofar as industrialism aims at mastering nature, it is bound to fail. This is not because the problems it creates are all insoluble. But there are no solutions which will not, in themselves, give rise to further problems. Moreover, many of them involve the mystery of human freedom and are therefore not, in a physical or mathematical sense, problems.

The idea of destiny implies an underlying harmony of man and nature, for a destiny is not a mere aspiration. It is an ontological imperative and must therefore be consonant with nature. If a destiny is transcendentally given, it must be naturally possible. This is why humans should not aim at mastery over nature, or look on nature as merely a great store of raw materials. Rather they should in action strive to elicit the basic accord that an understanding of destiny and of natural potentialities would reveal. This would mean resisting the temptation to make nature a servant of pride and physical pleasure and striving instead to bring forth the truth of nature, the comprehensive logos which harmonizes nature and humanity.

Our opposition to nature is so habitual that talk of an underlying harmony of humanity and nature is apt to seem implausible. Art and literature, however, indicate that such talk is not untrue. An Impressionist landscape is a vivid intimation of a paradise found at the heart of being—a paradise gained neither, as in pastoral dreams, by abstinence from action nor, as in capitalist and Marxist dreams, by triumphant action. Great poetry can arouse our consciousness of a physically manifest order grounded neither in pristine nature nor in industrial artifice, but in destiny. And the best architecture—say, a house designed by Frank Lloyd Wright—can awaken us to a fundamental accord between human beings and the natural universe. One of the principal functions of art is to establish a consciousness of this accord. The ugliness wrought by industrialism is not merely unpleasant. It is a sign of the violence we have done to nature, and it tends to stifle the sense of reality needed for subordinating industrial power to destiny.

Distant though it may be from typical attitudes of the present day, the idea that the human and the natural are in fundamental accord is one of the major themes in the philosophical traditions of the West. In the philosophies of Plato and Aristotle the supreme task of a human being is to ascend intellectually to ultimate being, to apprehend the logos governing at once the human and natural universe. Humanity is fulfilled in knowing and respecting a cosmic harmony that envelops both human beings and their physical surroundings. A sign of this harmony is found in the familiar, age-old idea of natural law; the moral and the natural in their depths are at one. The consonance of man and nature has been as prominent in religion as in philosophy. For the ancient Hebrews the physical universe reflected the purposes of the omnipotent Creator who brought forth men and women as well as light and sky, sea and land, fish, birds, and "beasts of the earth." This faith, against the powerful opposition of Manichean and Gnostic Christians, was incorporated in Christianity. Further, in Christian faith, the physical universe is dignified not only by its divine origins but also by the Incarnation. God's manner of redemption sanctified the human body. In the Gospel of John physical realities like bread, wine, and water are luminous symbols of spiritual realities. Even death, according to this consensus, does not necessarily signify the defeat of man by nature. For both Socrates and Paul, and for Plato as for Augustine, death could be, rather than a final blow dealt by fateful nature, an event within a personal destiny.

Fate and the Earth

Both Hebrews and Greeks in ancient times were more sensitive to the earth than is modern man, in his industrial pride. They were aware that human life, even in its most exalted forms, must have an appropriate physical setting. Thus in Hebrew scripture, the Christian Old Testament, "the earth is the Lord's and the fullness thereof." Through the earth humanity is related to the Creator, whose faithfulness "reaches unto the clouds," whose righteousness is "like the great mountains," whose "way is in the sea."[8] Upon the earth humanity has access to its destiny, and Job can say, "Speak to the earth and it shall teach thee."[9]

For the peoples of ancient Greece, the polis provided a uniquely suitable sphere for the realization of destinies. While the polis was not a purely natural setting, neither was it purely artificial. With its temples, civic buildings, marketplaces, and dwellings it provided a visibly human environment; but unlike the modern city, it was small, unpaved, and close to the countryside. Many citizens were farmers and much of life even inside the city was carried on out-of-doors. The Athenian Assembly met on an open hillside, judicial and commercial proceedings were often conducted in unsheltered public places, and philosophical inquiries were pursued in the sunlight of the agora. The earthliness of the polis was movingly evoked by Alfred Zimmern when he wrote of how "the Athenian had loved the Acropolis rock while it was still rough and unlevelled, when the sun, peeping over Hymettus, found only ruddy crags and rude Pelasgian blocks to illumine," and how he loved it even more "when its marble temples caught the first gleam of the morning or stood out, in the dignity of perfect line, against a flaming sunset over the mountains to the West."[10]

The Athenian Acropolis, with its marble temples, exemplifies the concept of the earth: neither untouched by humanity nor molded in every detail; rather, nature understood as a scene fitted for the enactment of destinies and thus crowned with emblems of humanity and of transcendence. Our situation in the twenty-first century is disturbing partly because of the state of the earth. Few of us see it habitually and frequently in its fusion of human and transcendental significance, as did many among the ancient Hebrews and Greeks; all of us see it at times ruthlessly violated; and most of us, enclosed in a purely artificial world, hardly see it at all.

In short, our physical surroundings have become reflective of fate. This results, as we have already seen, from a will to mastery in combination with the incapacity for mastery that is inherent in our finitude. We can of course scientifically understand limited segments of the physical universe, and accordingly we can shape limited areas of the earth in conformity with prior design. We can build beautiful parks and civic centers. But the physical universe as a whole evades our understanding, and accordingly the physical environment evades our control. The consequences are familiar to everyone.

There is, for example, the ugliness characteristic of large urban areas and of most industrial settings. A great art critic argues that beauty, by facilitating the act of perception, instills a consciousness of power.[11] Ugliness, conversely, brings feelings of weakness. If beauty testifies to an ontological harmony calling us to live a certain kind of life, then ugliness marks an encirclement by fate. A human race bent on industrial mastery necessarily cares little for beauty, and the unsightly surroundings it creates say nothing to us of destiny and confirm the state of mind, the disrespect for physical reality, in which they originate. It is noteworthy that the most appalling scenes of industrial squalor and desolation have been created by Communist nations, where the will to mastery and the scorn of transcendence was at its height, rather than in nations where such attitudes were moderated by religious traditions.

Another elemental and telling sign of our relationship to the earth can be seen in the dirt and poison that abound in our air, water, and food. Our physical surroundings are not altogether supportive even of life, to say nothing of destiny. This is because contaminating the environment is sometimes difficult to avoid and often profitable. Finitude and avarice conspire together. Destiny provides the form for life and hence as we abandon our concern for destiny we necessarily lose our ability to care for life. This is at least one source of the irony that we are surrounded by miracles of industrial mastery but often lack good water and healthful air.

Even if our surroundings were beautiful and healthful, however, it would be disturbing for them to be, as they are, continually and unpredictably changing. Human beings need things around them that are not merely familiar but are resonant with voices from the past. Thus T. S. Eliot, invoking our need for continuity, speaks of "a lifetime burning in every moment" and adds, "And not the lifetime of one man only/But of old stones that cannot be deciphered."[12] Those old stones speak of destiny and make up an essential part of the earth, properly understood. In our time they are too often torn up or covered over in the name of technological and industrial progress. Thus even one who resists the tides of mobility that engulf modern populations and spends a lifetime in one place may, due to a continually shifting physical environment, suffer from the uneasiness of the newcomer. The irony of fate is dramatically illustrated by our deprivation, in an age of large and dramatic physical undertakings, of so elemental a value as a firm and tranquil earth.

Fate and Death

Nature is threatening in various forms we have given it, such as the ugly and noxious physical settings many inhabit. It is more than threatening in a form we have not given it and cannot essentially alter, that of death. Here the whole human drive toward mastery comes to an unsuccessful end.

But is it an unsuccessful end? Modern man is fully cognizant of the denouement lying before him and does not appear greatly shaken. That

the life we have here on earth is the only life we shall ever have is
axiomatic in modern consciousness, at least so far as that consciousness
is defined by academicians, journalists, writers, and those who staff and
control the mass media. Most people, however, avow that the finality
of death in no way weakens their belief in life or their fidelity to the
altruistic morality that has for two millennia been linked with the idea
of personal immortality. Some assert even that the value of life is enhanced by the prospect of its obliteration and that morals are purified
by their separation from calculations of eternal reward. The modern
sense of mortality seems free of cynicism and despair.

Does the nonchalant bearing of modern man before "the king of
terrors" constitute a triumph of modern humanism, or is it a sign of
superficiality that we make so little of the brutal ascendancy that nature
will someday assert over each one of us? The question is not whether
life without hope of immortality must be terrifying or unhappy. It need
not be. Life has pleasures and joys that are not necessarily banished by
awareness of their evanescence. The question is not how we happen to
feel before the prospect of complete extinction but what we should
think. It is a question of logical implications. What is the meaning for
life of the finality of death?

A great writer of modern times has devoted much of his work in
one way or another to this question and has given an answer which for
me is fully convincing. The writer is Dostoevsky. The answer may be
summed up in the concept of demoralization. Dostoevsky saw modern man losing his Christian faith and in consequence facing, perhaps
in criminal or revolutionary self-assertion, perhaps in dissipation and
despair, the apparent certainty of complete personal annihilation. One
cannot live in a truly human way without respect for others and respect
for oneself, that is, without love. The comprehensive respect which is
love, however, is dependent on faith in the peculiar glory inherent in
personal immortality. When that faith disappears the result is demoralization, a state ensuing upon a twofold loss: of morality and of morale.

The loss of morality foreseen by Dostoevsky was expressed in his
well-known assertion that if death is final, "all is permitted." If every
reality is at last completely extinguished and forgotten, if every act and
event leads finally into oblivion, then it does not matter how we live.
Some, from native kindliness, perhaps, or from natural timidity, may
continue to obey the old Christian code. Others, however, differing in

temperament or circumstances, may not. Given the axiom that death is final, what can be said to them? Won't death, annihilating the criminal and tyrant (as well as the saint and martyr) and obliterating every trace and memory of their misdeeds, effectively clear the books? It is often said that people do not need to be lured or frightened by pictures of everlasting bliss or misery into behaving decently. Considering how indecently so many in our time have behaved, the validity of this contention is not evident. Dostoevsky's views are unfairly coarsened, however, if the issue be wholly reduced to that of whether humans will behave morally except under threat of eternal punishment. The issue is more sweeping and concerns the kind of spiritual crisis suggested by the word "nihilism." The moral devastation inherent in the belief that death is final is associated with the realization that if all realities and values are destined to disappear and be forgotten, then even now they are enveloped in a cosmic, irresistible indifference. A criminal or a tyrant—like a righteous man—is only an ephemeral appearance on the face of everlasting darkness. The consequences of every deed will trickle into historical rivers and thence into a sea of total oblivion.

It must be remembered how much Judaic-Christian morality demands of us: not just decency in our relations with those around us but rather treatment of every person according to the principle that a human being is of measureless worth. Raskolnikov was not inconsiderate of relatives and friends. He was not, in the ordinary sense of the word, selfish, nor was he unconcerned with the welfare of the human race. He was merely prepared to measure the worth of an old woman. And why not, if death is final? Morality rests in two ways on the premise of personal immortality. First, it depends on the faith that human beings are not mere passing phenomena; that is why their worth cannot be measured. Raskolnikov could tell himself that the old woman was of no use to society and hence of no value at all; and, physically spent, she would soon be dead even if she did not die at Raskolnikov's hands. Further, morality rests on the realization that, if I have offended against the moral law, I will be called to account, regardless of death. Mortality is not impunity.

Dostoevsky did not see the danger as solely that of unleashed selfishness, however. Those no longer in awe of eternity will not necessarily seek pleasure and advantage for themselves. On the contrary, they may try to redeem the world. And in their more grandiose and "selfless" undertakings they may be at their most murderous—an idea to which the Communist revolutions of the twentieth century lend sombre plausibility. Raskolnikov's ultimate aim—like Stalin's (assuming the sincerity of his Marxist professions)—was the happiness of the whole human race.

The other aspect of demoralization, loss of morale, may be understood simply as radical discouragement before the prospect of personal extinction. If one's being is defined not merely by the past and present but by all that one is yet to become—as the concept of destiny implies— then, if one is bound to become nothing, even one's past and present are nullified by mortality. Death does not wait at the end but reaches back and embraces the whole of life.

Loss of morale may also be understood, however, as resulting from the loss of morality. To be freed from all moral restraints does not place one in a state of glorious liberty. It threatens despair. If there is no reason for living in one way rather than another, life becomes a matter of whim and preference, without meaning. Morality is often spoken of as if it were a set of prohibitions that happen to be obligatory but impede the enjoyment of life. But the truth is that morality is recognition of the meaning of life in the form of imperatives of conduct. A life without such imperatives is without meaning and can hardly be enjoyable in any significant sense of the term. Hence the issue for Dostoevsky was not only how, in a universe ruled by death, we could live without scandalously misbehaving, but how we could live at all and not be overwhelmed by the absurdity of existence.

Morality, then, undergirds morale. But the converse also is true. When morale is lost, morality necessarily suffers. Those facing the apparent absurdity of existence will be less inclined than ever to adhere to the moral law. They may subside into peaceful but irresponsible apathy, or they may seek self-forgetfulness and a meaningful life in fanaticism.

From here, every road leads to tyranny. One motive is to escape from a freedom which is burdensome because life offers no meaningful choices. Another motive is order. When voluntary restraint ceases to exist, forcible restraint must take its place. And yet another motive is renown. Those whose thirst for immortality is not quenched metaphysically may try to satisfy it politically. A contemporary psychiatrist sees in the life of Mao Tse-tung a quest for "revolutionary immortality."[13] Hitler designated his regime a "Thousand-Year Reich." The multitudes who must serve as the raw materials for such projects, each one of them seen as fated for eventual extinction, cannot arouse moral inhibitions in the tyrant any more than can the blocks of marble with which he builds architectural and sculptural memorials of his power.

Modern man assumes that in believing in the finality of death he is only facing facts. But while death is a fact, its finality is not. It is mere assumption and surmise, plausible to people steeped in science and technology, but lacking the support even of the potent texts underlying the faith in personal immortality. Hence a question concerning motives is in order. To equate death with total extinction may sometimes be an act of courage, an adherence to apparent truth in spite of all personal longings. But it may often be a less creditable act than that. It may be an effort, not to face a hard truth, but to evade a disturbing one. Anticipation of eternal life is not necessarily a source of unalloyed comfort. The thought that there is no escaping from accountability for one's acts gives life a disquieting seriousness. It precludes comfortable and unconcerned enjoyment of the present moment. The modern sense of mortality is allied with our unapologetic devotion to pleasure and recreation.

It is allied also with pride. To affirm personal immortality is to associate every human being with a rationally impenetrable mystery. A being destined for eternal life cannot be totally accessible to rational investigation or designed management. Hence pride arouses resistance to the idea of personal immortality and inclines us to see human beings as objects and nothing more. Our certainty of death's finality thus is not necessarily a reasoned conclusion or a compelling intuition. It may be only a postulate required by our aspiration to universal dominion. This is not to suggest that all of this is plain in our minds. I mean only to point to the probability that our powerful will to mastery affects our conception of the reality to be mastered. If this is so, however, then it is the irony of our fate that the quest for boundless mastery has brought us to assumptions that imply our complete extinction.

We must bear in mind, therefore, that the defeat we face in having to die may not be a defeat inflicted by nature in itself but by nature transformed by human will into fate. Every human being has to die, but not every human being is *fated* to die. For some, death is destiny rather than fate. Although it is difficult to say exactly what this means, it is a matter of common experience. We all are aware of deaths, like those of Socrates and Jesus, that define and give meaning to life. But for people who have repudiated destiny in a drive toward dominion, death comes as an annihilating blow of fate. It is nature's final and unanswerable rejoinder to our pride.

The torments of our century, representing the irony of fate, have brought us to a crisis of the will. Facing a recalcitrant earth and finding ourselves in opposition to our own ideals, we experience deep frustration. The proposition that man is inhuman to man is a commonplace. Modern experience discloses a more complicated and trying truth: that the inhumanity of modern man comes from a sincere, if arrogant, effort to be human. It comes from an effort to humanize the earth and to liberate humanity. The crisis toward which yearning for sovereignty over the earth and history has led is reached when it becomes apparent that we must either give up the ideal of sovereignty or else, in one final surge toward dominion, set aside every limitation upon the will. This crisis can be described in terms of a simple alternative—receptivity or nihilism.

Epilogue: The True Political Art

When fate is ascendant, ordinary, democratic politics will seem ineffectual and barren. If events are hopelessly out of control, governing is necessarily a useless activity and is bound to be dispiriting. Those involved in it may be more than ordinarily inclined to counterbalance the frustrations inherent in their tasks with the gratifications of wealth and power, however dishonestly gained.

Our situation and state of mind today are not unlike those of the Greeks after the downfall of the city-state. Now as then history seems lethal and incomprehensible. In Greece certain philosophers condemned political life because of the useless cares it entailed and urged people to "live unknown." One powerful school, the Epicurean, advised that life be devoted to pleasure, or at least to the minimization of pain. It might be said that present-day industrial societies are inhabited mainly by practicing Epicureans. Almost everyone is preoccupied with the satisfactions thought to be found in material abundance. The major public institutions scarcely pretend to fulfill any function except that of ministering to this preoccupation. Life is essentially private, as Epicurus said it should be. Correspondingly, many look on politics, in a mood of Epicurean disdain, as largely unrelated to serious human interests.

It would be a mistake to dismiss such attitudes as merely cynical or selfish, either among the avowed Epicureans of ancient times or among the tacit Epicureans of the present day. Epicurus was morally serious and highly civilized, and for many people of antiquity his doctrine was a sober and seemingly saving way of life. Anyone who considers even for a moment the ways in which modern governments have failed—for example, through costly ineptitude (exemplified by the futile but endless trench battles of World War I and by interwar economic chaos) and through murderous spiritual pretensions (as in Communist and Fascist regimes alike)—might admit that contemporary Epicureans are not wholly unreasonable. The history of the twentieth century (called by Elizabeth Bishop "the worst century so far") suggests a certain sanity in devoting oneself to the pleasures of private life.

Nonetheless, if destiny is not only intimately personal but also universally human, Epicurus cannot be right. I experience my own personal destiny not merely in company with others but as being, in some sense, the same destiny that others—my friends and my fellow citizens—must live. I may feel at crucial moments that I am living the destiny of the whole human race. Correspondingly, in entering into relations with others, not only do I see traces of destiny in their lives (especially in the lives of those I love and in the lives of great historical figures), but sometimes I see these other destinies as somehow my own. The supreme moral command is that of love for one's neighbor. Since love is the recognition of a destiny, and my neighbor can be anyone on earth, I must live my own personal destiny as universally human. There was a fatal incongruity in Epicurus's effort to give weight and significance to private life by ignoring the life of the world around. His outlook depended on a materialism which, by obscuring and devaluating interpersonal relations, drained life of true significance at the outset.

It follows that resisting fate and being open to destiny requires that one learn to think and to act not merely as a private individual but also as a member of the human race. Being fully human is different in essence, and not merely in degree, from being a deer or a chimpanzee or a dog. A deer can be fully a deer without being conscious of the deer population of the earth or of the problems commonly affecting deer.

Not so a human being. Our humanity is not a natural form, realized fully in every member of the species by becoming like every other member of the species. It is a matter of consciousness and responsibility. One must have a sense of what human beings all over the earth are doing and suffering. And one must be prepared to act in behalf of not just one's own survival or well-being, but of any who happen to fall within the scope of one's powers. This is to say, in a word, that one must become political.

I understand politics to be the conduct of our lives in common. It follows that a relationship with others that is comprehensive (with all human beings, on the basis of all major components of a good life) and responsible (prepared for choice and action wherever these are appropriate) is political. To cultivate a consciousness of global problems and of their historical dimensions and deliberately to assume a position in relation to these problems is to adopt a political stance. And to inquire into our common problems and to act upon or endure them, according to circumstances, and so far as possible in company with others, is to take part in politics. This does not necessarily mean holding office or working with organizations; serious conversation can be a political activity. Here everything depends on personal temper, skill, and situation. A governmental official whose thoughts were only of carrying out routine duties or of garnering personal honor would be nonpolitical; a janitor or schoolteacher whose daily tasks were fulfilled as acts of conscious participation in the affairs of common life would be political. What is crucial is inhabiting as articulately and deliberately as possible the entire human situation: being positioned inquiringly and communally in relation to the great problems of one's own historical era.

I grant that personal relationships of a kind that are cultivated in private life also are essential to our humanity. But these need to be in a global setting to possess their full moral significance. Even my most intimate relationships are fully realized only so far as they are with people whom I know, not only in their own peculiarities, but in their universal humanity. I grant too that awareness of my full humanity is cultivated in ways we do not ordinarily think of as political—for example, by travel and by enjoyment of art and literature. But like private relationships, such activities attain their full moral significance only by being synthesized in a consciousness of global humanity, of its ordeals and acts, and of my own consequent obligations. And I grant, finally, that the most unsparing battles against fate often go on in solitude and not in political gatherings. But the only victory in these battles is in discerning and pursuing a destiny that is universally human, ours as well as mine, and the only hopeful struggle against fate is carried on—perhaps in utmost solitude—on behalf of all.

Our present-day loss of political bearings and habits is a sign of our having been overwhelmed by fate. If we are to keep our footing, which is our accessibility to destiny, we must cultivate a political consciousness that is without fanaticism but is also, as a consciousness of common humanity, unyielding. The art of doing this is "the true political art."

This phrase originated with Socrates, who said that he himself was the only Athenian who practiced the true political art. Socrates lived amid a people absorbed as few peoples have been in political rivalries and plans. Socrates himself was hardly involved in politics of this sort at all. He cared nothing for official status and showed little interest in day-to-day political issues. Not only did he remain aloof from political struggles, he was viewed with mistrust by his fellow citizens. In what sense, then, can the conduct of his life be called a political art?

In Socrates' stance two characteristics, apparently antithetical, yet in truth interdependent, are dramatically evident. (It may help the reader see these characteristics as political and as pertinent in modern times to note that they pertain also to a familiar American political figure, Abraham Lincoln.) First, Socrates was in a sense a solitary figure, in spite of the fact that he devoted his mature life to conversation. He was set apart from his fellow citizens by a singularity every Athenian was conscious of. We can only think of him as living through the climax of his destiny alone, spending his last hours with friends, yet marked off from them not just by the proximity of his death but by the mystery of his motives and his incomprehensible cheerfulness. (Lincoln was odd in appearance and manner, ridiculed on every side, and inhabited depths that were sensed but not comprehended by some of those around him.) At the same time, Socrates was an eminently communicative man. His readiness to listen and speak was not merely an inclination or habit but came from the essence of his personality. His very destiny lay in dialogue. (Lincoln, although a war leader, presiding over a conflict rare in scale and ferocity, inhabited circumstances tragically antithetical to his sociable and compassionate temper.) To understand the true political art, we must envision these two characteristics combined.

The phrase "solitary communality" indicates succinctly the posture of a person awaiting destiny in the presence of fate. The phrase is paradoxical and suggests a difficult personal balance. But in a civilization aggressively social and organizational, while spiritually desolate, solitude and communality both are imperative and belong together. This will become apparent as we briefly examine each attitude separately.

The individual in the face of fate is solitary. Fate sets people apart from one another. It may bind them together in giant organizations but in doing this it equates them with what is calculable and manageable in their personalities and thus falsifies them, precluding communal relationships. It renders them, even if organizationally fused, fundamentally alone. This is an aspect of the irony of fate. Bureaucrats, business executives, party leaders, and other agents of fate aspire to unite people totally; in fact they divide them through the processes of objectification to which their aims commit them.

Nothing is worse in this situation than for individuals to convince themselves that some particular historical entity, such as a state or a party, provides a way of evading or conquering fate. To be available for a destiny, each one must accept and live through a solitary confrontation with fate. This means keeping all historical idols at a distance, entering into only the most guarded relationships with ideologies, leaders, and parties. It means uncompromisingly maintaining one's moral autonomy, refusing to allow any authority to preempt the continuing task—the Socratic task!—of moral reflection and decision. Some of the most moving examples of this resolute solitude are seen among dissidents, exiles, and political prisoners. But such conduct is not alone for those impelled to practice some dramatic form of dissent. No one can be faithful to a destiny in times when fate is ascendant without practicing some form of disengagement, even if this be done in ways so inconspicuous as to be hardly discernible to an observer.

Yet solitude does not preclude communality. Although Socrates was so defiant of reigning opinion that he finally provoked Athens to kill him, he was in his defiance invincibly communal. He manifested his independence in speech. He seemed to live only in conversation and established his identity through dialogue. To think of Socrates is to think of a man in public places, engaged in common inquiry. It is to think likewise of one who even in his private moments must often have carried on inner conversations in preparation for the public conversations he pursued in the agora.

One might object that while Socrates may have been communal, he was not political, and it is true that the issues concerning him were not those of public policy. Rather, they were issues of moral character—the nature of virtues like courage and friendship. But the unstated aim of Socrates' conversations was to show that his interlocutors, and all who governed and guided Athens, were morally ignorant—unacquainted with the good in its various forms—hence unequipped for true political life. For Socrates, political competence was based on moral understanding, and his conversations were political in that this understanding can be gained only by those who have been humbled by being deprived of their illusions. Socrates' political art consisted in educating people for communicative inquiry into common, or political, ends.

Solitude and communality, then, constitute a single stance—a communal readiness in opposition to fate. Solitude is dedication to possibilities of communication that are neglected or closed off by established social and political forms. In this way, solitude arises from communality. Through the absolute commitments often made and glorified in our time, a party or nation is treated as though it were a perfect community. Solitude thus is done away with; but so is communality, for idolatry replaces the attentiveness and availability that frame the only gateway into community. Solitude signifies a refusal to enter into fraudulent communities and is in that way a communal state.

The true political art is essentially knowing how to live within historical time in readiness for destiny. Fate is a derangement of historical time, and it has its source in the ambition to rise above and master the flow of events in which our lives are set. But since that ambition cannot be realized, events contradict intentions. History takes the form of fate. The true political art enables one to resist the urge to historical mastery, devoting oneself instead, like Socrates, to the discovery through dialogue of the Logos, or meaning, which gives rise to destiny. Certainly the survival of individuals in their full humanity will often be determined by their capacity for standing out against the incivility of their times. Perhaps the survival of civilization will be decided by such individuals—a saving remnant who will take on the responsibilities implicit in the true political art.

This art depends ultimately on one's capacity for a certain kind of love—independent and inquiring, and politically sensitive. "Because iniquity shall abound," Jesus said, looking toward the upheavals in which he expected history to end, "the love of many shall wax cold."[14] Almost everyone today has experienced how readily love—attentiveness toward human beings, openness toward transcendence—"waxes cold." Jesus added, however, that "he that shall endure unto the end, the same shall be saved." The true political art, it might be said, is the art of enduring unto the end. It is the art of resisting fate through love, thus waiting for the destiny that not only brings traces of meaning into history but also singles out individuals and saves them from fate.

Notes

1. Reinhold Niebuhr, *The Irony of American History* (New York: Charles Scribner's Sons, 1952), viii.

2. Feodor Dostoevsky, *Crime and Punishment*, trans. Jessie Coulson (New York: W. W. Norton, 1964), 67.

3. Jonathan Schell, *The Time of Illusion* (New York: Alfred A. Knopf, 1976), 6 (italics added).

4. Romans 5:3 (Revised Standard Version).

5. Boris Pasternak, *Doctor Zhivago* (New York: Pantheon, 1958), 500.

6. Galatians 2:20 (RSV).

7. Romans 8:28 (King James Version).

8. These phrases are found, respectively, in Psalms 24:1, 36:5, 36:6, and 77:19 (KJV).

9. Job 12:8 (KJV).

10. Alfred Zimmern, *The Greek Commonwealth: Politics and Economics in Fifth-Century Athens*, 5th ed. (London: Oxford University Press, 1931), 68.

11. Bernard Berenson, *The Italian Painters of the Renaissance* (London: Oxford University Press, n.d.).

12. T. S. Eliot, *Four Quartets*.

13. Robert Jay Lifton, *Revolutionary Immortality: Mao Tse-tung and the Chinese Cultural Revolution* (New York: Vintage Books, 1968).

14. Matthew 24:12–13 (KJV).

CHAPTER TWO

Kant on Human Dignity

SUSAN M. SHELL

*A man who sins deviates from the rational order and so loses
his human dignity insofar as a man is naturally free and an end
unto himself.*

Thomas Aquinas, *Summa Th.*, 2a2ae.64.3

What does it mean to speak of "human dignity" or the dignity of man
as man? The term dignity is from the Latin *dignitas*, which means
virtue or worthiness, or, alternatively, honorable office. *Würde,* the term
Kant uses to translate *dignitas,* calls to mind the English "worth" and
"worthy."[1] Dignity, in Latin usage, refers especially to that aspect of
virtue or excellence that makes one worthy of honor—which, as Aristotle put it, accompanies virtue as its crown. Dignity, then, refers both
to a kind of deserving and to something deserved. In the Middle Ages,
dignity came to be especially associated with rank or authority that borrows something from the dignity of Christ. The dignity of the monarch,
for example, referred particularly to that aspect of kingship which, surviving the body, passes from one living sovereign to another (as in the
phrase, "the king is dead; long live the king").[2] Dignity, so understood,
was precisely *not* shared by all men equally, though all men, including
sovereigns, could be said to share the dignity deriving from our rank
as humans.

Prior to Kant, discussions of human dignity drew mainly from two overlapping traditions, one rooted in the Bible (or revealed religion generally), the other from classical philosophy. For the first, man's dignity derives from his status as a creature made in the image of God (and/or reborn in Christ). For the other, man's dignity derives from his status as a rational being, able to contemplate nature and able to justify thereby the value of human existence. Philosophic reason and supraphilosophic (or nonphilosophic) revelation were, then, the twin pillars on which man's claims to dignity, or worthiness of honor and esteem, were largely set. Pico della Mirandola's famous *Oration on the Dignity of Man*, which locates human dignity in our freedom, is only an apparent exception to this rule. For the freedom of which della Mirandola speaks is ultimately guided, on his account, by theoretical knowledge (without which that freedom would be worthless). To be sure, della Mirandola's appeal to human excellence also calls to mind poetic treatments of the ancient heroes, for whom honor is a matter of distinction and hence inherently unequal.

Kant's treatment of human dignity is something new. To be sure, his discussion has something in common with the traditions that precede it. Like the ancient philosophers, he links dignity with reason;[3] and like the theologians he finds its deepest source in what we share as creatures who must choose rather than in natural endowments that lift some above others. Finally, like the ancient poets, Kant imbues dignity with a kind of heroism, as in his definition of virtue as spiritual courage. Still, his treatment is more than a (more or less consistent) borrowing from these earlier sources. Man is exalted, for Kant, neither by nature nor by God, as classical philosophy and biblical religion respectively insist, nor by the martial glory celebrated by the ancient poets, but by autonomy, or subjection to self-made law, as announced and certified by conscience.[4]

One gets some sense of the personal transformation that led Kant to this insight (and to which he wished to guide others) from a famous confessional note, set down when he was about forty, which sets the value of cosmological inquiry against that deriving from what we share as humans.

I am by nature an inquirer. I feel a whole thirst for knowledge and a desirous restlessness to come into more of it, along with satisfaction in each acquisition. There was a time when I thought that this alone could constitute the honor of mankind, and I despised the people [*Pöbel*] who know nothing. Rousseau brought me to rights [*hat mich zurecht gebracht*]. This imaginary prejudice vanished, I learned to honor human beings [*Menschen*], and I would find myself less useful than the ordinary worker if I did not believe that this consideration could give value to all the others, in establishing [*herzustellen*] the rights [*Rechte*] of humanity [*Menschheit*].[5]

Biographically speaking, Kant's moralized understanding of human dignity goes together with a doctrine of equal rights understood not as a fact of nature (as with Hobbes and Locke) but as an ideal, i.e., something that needs to be historically established because it *ought* to be.

In Kant's later thought, this transformation persists, as we shall see, in his understanding of respect (rather than benevolence or love) as the primary quality of a morally good attitude. Treating human beings as ends in themselves implies above all treating them as fellow end-setters who I am not permitted to affect by my actions other than in ways that they (actively or passively) consent to.[6]

Dignity and Autonomy

Dignity, on Kant's account, adheres to us by virtue of "moral personality," or "the freedom of a rational being under moral laws." ("Psychological personality," on the other hand, is "the capacity for being conscious of one's identity in different conditions of one's existence.")[7] A "person" in the moral sense is thus "a subject whose actions can be *imputed* to him," which implies that he is free. Freedom, as Kant famously puts it, is the *ratio essendi* of the moral law; while conscience, or our awareness of the moral law, is the *ratio cogniscendi* of freedom. Freedom, in other words, is the ground or reason without which there would not be a moral law, while awareness of the moral law, or conscience, is the ground or reason for our recognizing that we are free. ("Ought," in short, implies "can.")

But how does one get from moral freedom in general to autonomy, such that (as Kant concludes) "a person is subject to no law other than those he gives himself" (alone or with others)? Kant's reasoning is roughly as follows: only by virtue of autonomy, or subjection to self-made law, can the practical necessity that characterizes the moral law's categorical command be reconciled with the freedom to obey to which the moral law also immediately testifies [VI 223; 49–50]. That the moral law (like the content of empirical experience) is given, and yet (unlike empirical experience) is necessary rather than contingent, points to its special character as a "fact of *reason* [emphasis added]," and, indeed, the only fact of this nature:

> Consciousness [of the moral law] may be called a fact of reason, since one cannot ferret it out [*herausvernünfteln*] from any antecedent data of reason, . . . and since it forces itself upon us as a synthetic a priori proposition. . . . In order to regard this law without any misinterpretation [*Mißdeutung*] as *given*, one must well note: that it is not empirical but the sole fact of reason by virtue of which "[reason] announces itself as originating law [*ursprünglich gesetzgebend*] (*sic volo, sic jubeo*)."[8]

Autonomy, on this account, follows immediately from the categorical nature of morality's demands. The moral law, which is "given" and yet necessary (rather than contingent, as is the case with all empirically "given" facts), must, *as* necessary, originate in reason.[9] Interpreted aright, the moral law not only "forces itself" upon us but also "announces" its own autonomous foundation.

Autonomy of the will—the "sole principle of all moral laws" [V 32; 33]—belongs, then, not only to the virtuous, but to all "persons," by which Kant means "beings to whom actions can be imputed." Dignity, in short, applies to any finite being who has, or can be presumed to have, a conscience. It is thus something that all human beings possess because we are all co-legislators of the moral law. (Degree does not enter in here, since to be accountable in any way is to be free in the morally decisive sense and hence infinitely raised about anything [else] in nature.) It is true that Kant speaks of certain vices (e.g., lying) as a kind of forfeiture, or "throwing away," of one's humanity. At the same time, for Kant, there is no action we can take that altogether destroys the possibility of moral improvement, now or in the future, and hence no annihilation of our moral personality in any absolute sense.

Whatever has reference to universal human inclinations and needs has a market price; whatever, without presupposing a need, accords with a certain taste, i.e., a delight in the mere unpurposive play of our forces of soul [*Gemüthskräfte*], has an affective price [*Affectionspreis*]; but that which alone constitutes the condition under which something can be an end in itself does not have a merely relative value [*Werth*], i.e., a price, but rather an inner value, i.e., a dignity [*Würde*].[12]

Our estimation of virtue, and humanity insofar as it is capable of it, "puts it infinitely beyond all price" with which morality "cannot be brought into competition" without, as it were, "violating its sanctity."[13]

Morality is thus the vehicle through which we participate in an economy of absolute value—an "intelligible world" whose necessitating bonds affirm our irreplaceability, and thus "reveal" a life, on our part, "beyond all sense"—despite the humiliating fact, to which human consciousness also testifies, that as beings of need we are fated to arise and perish. As Kant famously states at the conclusion of the *Critique of Practical Reason:*

Two things fill the mind [*Gemüth*] with ever new and increasing admiration [*Bewunderung*] and awe [*Ehrfurcht*] the oftener and more steadily we occupy ourselves with reflecting on them: the starry heaven above me and the moral law within me. Both I do not merely conjecture as obscured in darkness or in the transcendent [*Überschwenglichen*] exceeding my circle of vision; I see them before me and they connect immediately with consciousness of my existence. The former begins at the place that I occupy in the external world of sense, and it extends the connection in which I stand into an unbounded [*unabsehlich*] magnitude of world beyond worlds. . . . into the limitless times of their periodic motion, their beginning and their continuance. The latter begins at my invisible self, my personality, and exhibits me in a world that has true infinity, but which is traceable only by the understanding—and a world with which I recognize myself in a connection that is not merely contingent but universal and necessary. The former view of countless multitudes of worlds annihilates, so to speak, my importance, as an animal creature that must give back to the planet (a mere speck in the universe [*Weltall*]) the matter from which it came, the matter that is for a little time provided (we know not how) with vital force. The latter, on the contrary, lifts up [*erhebt*] my value [*Werth*] as an intelligence by my personality, in which the moral law reveals [*offenbart*] a life independent of animality, and even of the entire sensible world—at least insofar as it allows itself to be assumed from the purposive determination of my existence [*Dasein*] through this law, which is not bounded by the conditions and limits of this life, but goes [on] into the infinite.[14]

Dignity, for Kant, is, then, connected with a kind of immortality beyond temporal calculation in an everyday sense.[15] Human consciousness testifies both to our location in a world informed by space and time (whose "ideality" *The Critique of Pure Reason* is devoted, in part, to establishing) and to a status that transcends it.

Kant's famous evocation of the sublimity of the moral life—all the more striking in its contrast with the (related) awe [*Ehrfurcht*] inspired by our position in the natural universe—is, in at least one respect, however, ambiguous: human dignity as a subjective feeling of being "lifted up" involves our simultaneous awareness of ourselves as spectator/ participants in the world (in which our value is virtually zero) and as (priceless) legislators of a world beyond—"in so far as the purposive determination of one's existence through this law may be assumed." But on what ground does that assumption rest? Does the moral law suffice? Or is other, worldly evidence required (as Kant's language equally suggests)? Can we, in short, truly *feel* our elevation without further assurance that humanity's worldly existence somehow counts? Kant's equivocation puts us on alert concerning the possible importance of history (or the purposive determination of our existence in *this* world) to a subjective appreciation of man's worth.

Reason and End-Setting

The moral law allows understanding to trace the form of an intelligible world in which we too participate, but not the content, which would require an immediate intuition (accessible to God alone) of the reality of freedom. Our task, according to Kant, is, rather, to actualize the intelligible world in the here and now (to the extent that it is possible), and thereby bring the "two standpoints" of human consciousness—incommensurable and yet somehow united—into ever greater harmony or attunement. But this, in turn, means bringing freedom and law into outward harmony (since inner harmony eludes our intuitive grasp) of a sort that makes consent a condition of all (other) ways that I may permissibly affect someone.

This understanding of reason sheds light on Kant's famous insistence that one "treat humanity,[16] whether in one's own person, or the person of another, not only as a means but also as an end [or 'end in itself']."[17] This injunction requires, above all, that we respect man's status as a rational being, i.e., a being (the only one we know of) who not only can be an end (in the sense of serving as a means, either to himself or others) but who can also (lawfully) set or have an end. To have an end—a goal, consciously before one—is, finally, to set it for *oneself*, on the basis of one's own reason.

Reason, according to Kant, is less a faculty of knowledge than a capacity to project or originate "ideas" that possess regulative or practical necessity—less about what is than about what should be. Leaving aside the (hypothetical) case of God—the divine intellect that knows what it creates—reason's ideas are best understood not as objects of an immediate theoretical intuition of reality (as Platonism, according to Kant, wrongly maintains) but as foci (as in *focus imaginarius*) of reason's self-imposed, rule-governed demands. Reason, in short, is essentially a capacity for self-necessitation, or the setting for oneself of binding tasks. In the case of its theoretical employment, in the service of attaining knowledge of the natural world (or, as Kant would say, the world as it appears to us), this demand takes the form of a striving toward totality (or self-consistent, all-embracing unity) as directed by the "regulative" goal of perfect knowledge of nature as a whole. We do not directly intuit such a whole (and, given the finitude of human reason, never will), but we do strive, according to Kant, in all our scientific undertakings to approach what thereby serves us as a "regulative" goal. (Hence, the crucial role of "ideas" in defining what it is to be a science.) This understanding of ideas rests, to be sure, on a "critique" of reason's claims to knowledge of a sort to which Platonism, according to Kant, pretends and that an equally misguided skepticism altogether disallows.

The details of this critique, which take up many pages of Kant's *Critique of Pure Reason*, cannot detain us here. It is enough, for our purposes, to underscore the extent to which reason, for Kant, ceases to be, primarily, a vehicle of theoretical knowledge without ceasing thereby to be something ordinary understanding deems, or can identify as, rational. At least since the time of Aristotle, the rule against self-contradiction and the hope if not the certainty that reason suffices as a guide to what is good have defined the basis of the rational or philosophic life. All that Kant removes is the belief or expectation that at the highest level this guidance takes the form of theoretical knowledge (as distinguished from "revelation" through the moral law). Reason's self-critique (for that is what Kant claims his argument to be) not only drives home the fallacy of such expectations, conducive as they are to self-contradiction, which, in the case of conflict between the principle of freedom and that of natural necessity (the "third cosmological antinomy") bears especially hard on moral life. It also exhibits the sufficiency of reason to serve as its own self-judging and self-correcting tribunal. Both directly and indirectly, then, the critique of pure reason affirms the autonomy of reason (and with it the formula of humans as ends-in-themselves) to which conscience bears witness by a different route.

Implications of Kant's Conception of Human Dignity for Ethics and Politics

Kant's association of human dignity with our status as imputable end-setters forms the basis of a discussion of human rights and virtues that fills out the formal contours of the categorical imperative: "act only on the basis of maxims that you can at the same time will to be universal law."

Whereas reason in its theoretical employment is directed by the idea of nature as totality, it is guided in its practical employment by the Idea of the "Highest [moral] Good"—or virtue (i.e., worthiness to be happy) and happiness combined. (Even a perfectly holy and omnipotent being, reason can confidently assert, could intuit nothing better.) Since we cannot make others virtuous nor avoid intending our own happiness, the idea of the highest good issues in broad, positive duties to perfect ourselves and to promote the happiness of others, leaving it to God (and, in a qualified sense, to history) to bring the distribution of virtue and happiness into just proportion.

The collective nature of the end of moral legislation subordinates itself, however, to the individual nature of the wills in which the law itself originates. Humanity, for Kant, precisely because of its nonfungibility, is never reduced to a collective subject. (For Kant, unlike the infamous aparatchik in Arthur Koestler's *Darkness at Noon*, future flower gardens do not and cannot justify present massacres.) The "narrow" and "perfect" negative duty to refrain from using humanity in my own person or that of another merely as a means trumps the "wide" and "imperfect" positive duty to perfect myself or benefit others.

What does it mean to refrain from using humanity in my own person as a mere means? To begin with, this duty implies that I may not use my own reason, or lawmaking and end-setting power, to serve natural inclinations that ought, properly, to be reason's tool. According to Kant, mutilating oneself either temporarily (he cites, e.g., birth control) or permanently (e.g., suicide) is to deprive oneself of the "natural" (and so indirectly the moral) use of one's powers, and, in so doing, "to root out the existence of morality itself in this world so far as one can."[18] To respect humanity in one's own person is thus to acknowledge certain natural limits, implicit in our organic constitution, to which our body may properly be put. Recognition of such limits does not rest on claims to theoretical knowledge of natural purposes (as with Aristotle) but on an immediate awareness of ourselves as living beings in the world, however much that status may defy final empirical explanation. Hence the ascendance of freedom over nature does not, for Kant, authorize using one's body in ways that conflict with its own, self-organizing tendencies, except in those cases where duty itself requires one to risk one's life or health. To respect humanity in my own person is to acknowledge a certain naturally purposive (but nonhierarchical) order of the body, which supports rational activity without defining it. *Bildung* in the sense of education presupposes, without being directed by, *Bild* in the sense of natural form: the imperfect duty to cultivate my skills (which can proceed in a variety of ways) bows before the perfect duty not to abuse the organism in which my moral life, in this world at least, necessarily takes shape. Readers more familiar with the work of later thinkers who claim Kantian provenance may be surprised at the severity of his views on issues such as birth control and bodily mutilation, both of which he ethically (but not legally) condemns. The point here is not whether or not Kant's particular views on these matters are correct, but the robust connection between human dignity, as Kant conceives it, and the link between the "two standpoints of *embodied* rationality" (from which we respectively reflect upon the starry heavens above and the moral law within)—a link that somehow unifies these vantage points without collapsing them.

Man's duty to himself as a moral being *only*, on the other hand, has to do with "what is *formal* in the harmony [*Übereinstimmung*] of the maxims of his will with the *dignity* of humanity in his person" and consists in prohibitions against lying, avarice, and false humility. These vices "adopt principles that are directly contrary" to "inner freedom," and hence "the innate dignity of man," which is as much as to say that they "make it a principle to have no basic principle and hence no character" [VI 420; 216–17]. The liar, for example, makes himself "less even than a thing," for a thing, being "real and given, has the property of being serviceable, so that another can put it to some use."[19]

> But communication of one's thoughts through words that yet (intentionally) contain the contrary of what the speaker thereby thinks, is a posited [*gesetzter*] end directly opposed to the natural purposiveness of one's power of communicating one's thoughts, and [as such] a renunciation of one's personality, and a mere deceptive appearance of a man rather than a man himself.[20]

Avarice and false humility involve a similar failure to treat one's person as a purposive whole (at least potentially), informed by rational ends. Avarice, for its part, is a refusal to make use of means in one's possession for enjoying life, so as to leave one's true needs unsatisfied (VI 433; 229), while servility or false humility involves a failure to insist upon the value of one's person in comparison with others.

> In the system of nature man (*homo phenomenon, animal rationale*) is a being of slight importance and shares with the rest of the animals, as offspring of the earth, a common value (*pretium vulgare*). Although man has, in his understanding, something more than they and can set himself ends, even this gives him only an *external* value

(*pretium usas*); that is to say, it gives one man a higher value than another, that is, a *price* as a commodity in exchange with these animals as things, though he still has a lower value than the universal medium of exchange, money, the value of which can therefore be called preeminent (*pretium eminens*).

But man considered as a *person* . . . is lifted up [*erhaben*] above all price; for as a person (*homo noumenon*) he is not to be valued merely as a means to the ends of others or even to his own ends, but as an end in himself; that is, he possesses a *dignity* (absolute inner value) by which he necessitates *respect*.

Humanity in one's person is thus

the object of a respect that one can demand from every other man, but which one also must not forfeit. . . . Since one must regard oneself not only as a person in general but also as a human being, i.e., as a person who has duties laid upon him by his own reason, one's insignificance as a human animal [*Thiermensch*] must not do damage [*Abbruch*] to one's consciousness of one's dignity as a rational man [*Vernunftmensch*] . . . [hence] one should pursue one's end, which is in itself a duty, not abjectly, not in a *spirit of servility* (animo servili) . . . but always with consciousness of the sublimity [*Erhaben-heit*] of one's moral predisposition (which is already contained in the concept of virtue). [21]

Proper humility, on the other hand, comes from a comparison of ourselves with the moral law in all its strictness, and thus entails exaltation (*Erhebung*) and the "highest self-esteem" for oneself in one's capacity as moral lawgiver. Respecting humanity in my own person thus also means not allowing myself to be used merely as means by others, even, and perhaps especially, when they do so on the basis of a claim to serve me. Asserting one's rights, even at risk of one's life, is, for Kant, a perfect duty, and never more so than when my very right to do so is itself at stake. (Although morality does not authorize violent revolution, something approaching enthusiasm[22] over the result is, for Kant, the one sure sign that "humanity is constantly progressing toward the better.")

For reasons that are not hard to see this principle, directed against paternalistic monarchs (who, from Kant's point of view, treat their subjects like sheep rather than human beings), assumes crucial, if not revolutionary, political importance.[23] The traditional justification of rule on the grounds that it benefits the ruled is here undone, not, as with Hobbes, because rulers cannot be trusted to serve others, but because the justification for ruling that they advance poses a direct challenge to man's status as a source, not just an object, of value.

The system of ethics (whose positive duties are benevolence and self-perfection) thus presupposes a system of rights that imposes absolute negative conditions on the actions I am morally allowed to undertake, be my ends morally proscribed, permitted, or forbidden. The liberal regime that Kant morally refounds does not justify itself in terms of human happiness but civic honor, however much concern for happiness can be counted on to help to realize it. Ulpian's "honeste vive"— live honorably—is the first rule, for Kant, of civic justice. (That the system of rights is supported by immoral as well as moral motives, and hence evinces the [fractured][24] purposiveness of our own nature, is a theme we shall return to.)

Rights, for Kant, have both a "private" and a "public" aspect. Rights in a private sense define a system of property law which, according to his famous formula, maximizes "the freedom of each consistent with the freedom of all the rest." By "freedom" Kant here means access, unobstructed by the will of others, to the use of objects as means. Subjection of that freedom to the condition that it coexist lawfully with the freedom of others means not using others (or what belongs to them) as means except in ways that they consent to. Kant's formula for civic justice thus approximates the workings of an ideal marketplace, whose outcomes are, by definition, the result of voluntary exchanges of property, itself acquired either through previous exchanges or "originally," i.e., through the appropriation of things not already owned.

Property in one's own body cannot be alienated, for reasons earlier suggested; otherwise everything in nature can be appropriated, either originally or by exchange. Hence we see once again the inseparability of human dignity in a Kantian sense and the market as a (an opposing) measure of value. The juridical community consists of persons, who may not be used against their will, and things, the use of which is otherwise unrestricted. (A variation—property in persons as if they were things—principally involves the sexual rights of spouses, which Kant derives from an idea of personal integrity, or wholeness, that forbids nonreciprocal consumption [through exhaustion or death in childbirth] of another's body.) Property for Kant does not belong to the person who can "use it well," nor does his juridical scheme recognize any prior articulation of the world according to purposes natural or divine.

To enjoy the civil status of a citizen (itself a "dignity" in the sense of honorable office) is to be formally free and equal and materially self-sufficient or capable of living off one's own property according to one's own direction (as distinguished from a wife, servant, day laborer, or pauper, all of whom depend for their livelihood on others who direct them). Kant's somewhat archaic understanding of economic self-sufficiency as a condition of civic equality can be brought closer in line with modern liberal sensibilities, if we reflect on Abraham Lincoln's hope that every citizen might, at some point in his life, work for himself rather than another.[25] Even in America today, "being one's own boss" holds an attraction for many that has less to do with a desire for security than with the respect that we collectively attach to what we (and Kant) call "standing on one's own two feet."

Public right, or government, is necessary, not only because individuals are ill-equipped to defend their rights on their own, but because they cannot do so without doing violence to their adversaries, whom they thereby treat as a mere means. Only the state is authorized to punish wrongdoers retributively (not just restrain them),[26] hence with a view to their imputability or inner freedom. Thus only the state can reconcile the need to cancel cancellations of freedom through the coercion of wrongdoers, actual or potential, with the duty to respect wrongdoers as persons.

The constitution in conformity with this end is republican in the precise sense of separating the power of making law—a power elected by the people—from the executive (and judicial) power that applies it. Not only is republicanism the only just form of government; it is, Kant goes so far as to say, the only form of government, lacking which there is no true civic body. Such a form ideally exists even in regimes that fall short of republicanism "in the letter," by virtue of the fact that they enforce rights, properly understood, to some degree, and do not in principle rule out the possibility of progress in actualizing the ideal. Deviations from pure justice (e.g., the feudal and absolutist regulations of Kant's Prussia) are permissible, so long as they are imposed in a way that leaves open hope in their eventual legal abolition, however temporally

remote. Given that hope, citizens are free to interpret the civic impediments from which they presently suffer as a prudential concession on
the rulers' part to current circumstances (be those concessions well- or
ill-advised), rather than as a principled assertion of his subjects' intrinsic
civic inferiority and/or idiocy.[27] That a ruler should, in principle, declare
his subjects altogether lacking in rights, so that his relation to them is
one of pure ethical benevolence (as with a shepherd and his sheep) is,
according to Kant, both morally and prudentially impossible—morally
so, because it reverses the relation between right and ethics on which
genuine morality depends, and prudentially so, because a people confronted with paternalism in so explicit and unambiguous a form would
certainly (or so Kant claims) revolt.[28]

History and the Collective Worth of Human Existence

Kant's renunciation of the traditional religious view as to the source of
human dignity—a view according to which the superiority of the origins goes without saying[29]—gives new moral urgency to the question
of human progress. "We can scarcely help feeling," Kant says,

> a certain distaste on observing [men's] activities as enacted in the
> great world-drama, for we find that, despite the apparent wisdom
> of individual actions here and there, everything as a whole is made
> up of folly and childish vanity, and often of childish malice and
> destructiveness. The result is that we do not know what sort of con-
> cept we should have of our species, which is so proud of its sup-
> posed superiority.[30]

The "only way out for the philosopher," is to seek to discover a "purpose in nature" behind the seemingly senseless course of human events.
Without some additional (historical) assurance as to the purposiveness
of mankind's collective existence here on earth, the tension—unreliev-
able in this life—between the I as worldly spectator and the I as moral
subject, a tension on which the *Critique of Practical Reason* insists, points
not to eternity (or to "that which, on account of its objective character,
exists necessarily, as the final purpose of an intelligent cause")[31] but to
our fractured nature and condition as a species.

But how to find a purpose in nature, when nature, as scientifically knowable, is devoid of purpose? Kant's *Critique of Judgment* finds an answer in the notion of "culture," or "man's aptitude [*Tauglichkeit*][32] in general for setting himself purposes, and for using nature ... as a means, in conformity with the maxims of his free purposes generally."[33] Culture, so defined, enables us to regard nature as a whole as purposive, so long as culture is subordinated to "man as moral subject," which Kant calls "the final purpose of creation itself."

The fulfillment of culture depends, in turn, upon the advent of republicanism: "The formal condition under which nature can alone achieve [its] final aim is that constitution of human relations where the impairment [*Abbruche*] which results from mutual conflicting freedom is countered by lawful authority in a whole, called civil society."[34] Man's "asocial sociability"—his crooked tendency, coeval with reason itself, to subjugate himself and others—culminates, on such a view, in free self-government, allowing for the full development of all men's faculties.

Although the passage to republicanism is fostered by man's asocial sociability, the process is not automatic: true, "the problem of politics can be solved for a nation of devils, if only they have understanding." Still, it cannot be solved *by* them.[35] Hence the need for the emergence of a saint/philosopher/king, or barring that near impossibility,[36] of otherwise arousing men's awareness of their honorable, and, indeed, sublime, vocation as self-legislating citizens—a task that epitomizes the calling of philosophy as Kant himself conceives it.

Events near the end of Kant's life (and connected with the French Revolution) called forth new efforts on his part to establish that mankind is "in constant progress toward the better." These efforts responded to a double fear: first, that the duplicitous benevolence of paternalistic monarchs might lead subjects of the most powerful European states to forgo their rights; second, that the same rulers might literally consume their subjects, along with the other peoples of the earth, in catastrophic wars.[37] In making his case, Kant sets the prospect of mankind's self-undoing against the fact of man's natural insignificance—a formulation that recalls the famous juxtaposition of the natural and moral sublime quoted earlier:

Before the omnipotence [*Allgewalt*] of nature, or even more, before its to us inaccessible highest cause, man is, in his turn, but a trifle

[*Kleinigkeit*]. But for the sovereigns [*Herrscher*] of his own species to take and treat him as such, in part by burdening him bestially, as mere tool of their intentions [*Absichten*], in part by exposing him in their conflicts with one another, in order to let him be slaughtered—that is no trifle, but an overturning [*Umkehrung*] of the ultimate purpose [*Endzweck*] of creation itself.[38]

Kant's bleakest thought is a future in which prospects for the civil condition are permanently darkened, forestalling the self-emancipation of humankind by submerging the principle of autonomy, and with it human dignity, in paternalistic oblivion.

Here, then, is a powerful reason for Kant's extraordinary claims on behalf of the "sympathy" aroused in "wishful spectators" of the French Revolution, a response that Kant deems a "sign," "never more to be forgotten," that "mankind is in constant progress toward the better."[39] For what this response signals, above all, is a representation of human history that unites the distinct moments of sublimity that *Critique of Practical Reason* consecutively evoked:[40]

> This event is the phenomenon, not of a revolution, but rather . . . of the evolution of a constitution according to natural right [*einer naturrechtlichen Verfassung*], which, to be sure, is still not itself to be achieved only by wild battles—for war destroys all previously standing inward and outward statuary constitutions—and which therefore leads to a striving after a constitution that cannot be bellicose, namely, a republican constitution. . . . Here, therefore, is a proposition that is not just well-meaning and commendable for a practical intention, but, despite all skeptics, maintainable for the most rigorous theory: that the human race has always been in constant progress toward the better and will continue to be henceforth; which, if one has regard not only for what happens to one people, but also to the extension [*Verbreitung*] [of that progress] over all peoples of the earth, who gradually come to participate in it, *opens/ inaugurates a prospect of incalculable time* [*die Aussicht in eine unabsehliche Zeit eröffnet*]. (Emphasis added)[41]

Kant's thesis, or the event securing it, opens up a prospect that combines the incalculability of the natural world with a glimpse of the eternal—a glimpse available to us by virtue of our higher, moral nature. Or it does so, as Kant continues, "insofar [*wofern*] that there does not, per chance, occur a second epoch of natural revolution which pushes aside [*mitspielen*] the human race to let other creatures strut upon the stage." And yet, by guaranteeing that men will not forever accept the deceptively benign blandishments of rulers, the event in question (or Kant's rendering of it) secures us from a feeling that would otherwise challenge (according to the terms laid down) moral sublimity itself, or "the uplifting of our value . . . above anything in nature."

So construed, Kant's concern with history is no mere afterthought, but the outcome of a conception of human dignity that relies, for its potency, not only on the moral law, but also on some assurance against despair, also morally derived, as to the pointlessness of our collective existence—a pointlessness that may finally put human dignity itself in question.[42]

Evaluation and Conclusion

How does Kant's idea of human dignity stand up to the alternatives mentioned at the beginning of this chapter? Kant's understanding of freedom as autonomy raises one obvious difficulty: how can we understand wrongdoing as free and yet contrary to the moral law? Kant deals with this difficulty, in part, by distinguishing *Wille*—that aspect of the soul which morally legislates—from *Willkür* (or freedom of choice), and, more generally, by drawing our attention to the divided nature of the moral self revealed by conscience, a self both humbled and exalted. If interpreting freedom as autonomy leaves mysterious the culpability of evil (or action that is free yet contrary to the moral law), this, in the end, is a problem that Kant is prepared to live with. The possibility of freedom (and hence of both good and evil) is finally incomprehensible, as he argues at the conclusion of the *Groundwork,* for finite minds like ours.[43] And in any case, Kant would say, it is better, from the standpoint of moral self-consistency, to accept the mysteriousness of evil than to endeavor to explain it on the basis of original sin—a notion that violates the fundamental moral principle that one is accountable only for one's own actions.[44]

Another potential criticism of Kant stems from the short shrift he gives to questions of relative rank and merit. (See especially the essay by Robert P. Kraynak, chapter 3 in this volume.) Honor, in the proper sense, for Kant, is always *honestas* or integrity, never *honor*, or distinction of a sort that lessens the honor owed to others. The Kantian understanding of human dignity diminishes (and means to diminish) our susceptibility to a kind of human excellence whose impressiveness is inseparable from elevation in rank above that of other human beings.[45] According to Kant, all persons are obliged to have and hence capable of goodwill—the one thing good without qualification that it is possible to think.[46] The only unqualified good is in this sense universally accessible.[47]

True, Kant's universalism is anything but easygoing. Virtue, for Kant, is a strenuous affair, requiring (uncommon) moral strength and fortitude.[48] Most difficult of all, it involves a never-ending effort to be truthful with oneself, lest one be reduced, in one's own eyes, to what Kant calls a "speech machine"—a mere "appearance" of a human being whose "determination" is so far from "purposive" as to be literally incapable of meaning anything.[49] (Such systemic and largely internal considerations may, indeed, have led Kant to exaggerate the significance of dishonesty beyond the limits of ordinary moral understanding.)[50] That all human beings deserve respect is not to say that "anything goes." Far from it, for a thinker for whom the goodness of happiness itself depends on our making ourselves worthy of it. It is, however, to say that moral judgment, in the strict sense, cannot be exercised toward others, whose inner motives are more hidden from us even than our own. (For reasons earlier suggested, Kant's treatment of civil punishment is only an apparent exception to this rule.) The temperamental baseline of Kant's worries about human dignity is less sanguine than melancholy—less "I'm OK, you're OK" than "judge not lest ye be judged." To put matters another way, the value of human life—both its goodness for us and our worthiness to enjoy it—is not, for Kant, a foregone conclusion. "The value of life," he once said, if it is lived for the sake of mere enjoyment (i.e., happiness) is easy to estimate: "it sinks below zero." "For who would enter life anew under the same conditions, or even under a plan he had devised for himself (though in conformity with the course of nature) but that aimed merely at enjoyment?"[51] Kant's affinity with earlier liberal notions of the imperviousness of the individual (within certain limits) to public scrutiny and condemnation has less to do with the weakening or abandonment of moral standards (of which earlier liberals are often accused) than with an internalization that boosts those standards beyond the limits of space and time (and, in this sense, infinitely raises them) with a concomitant devaluation of public, political life as the arena of a freedom that is "merely external." And yet public life, as the visible phenomenon of our moral relations with one another, remains the theater in which man's moral destiny, in this life, is necessarily played out—and upon which, as we have seen, the "revelation" of our dignity, for Kant, at least partly draws.

These strains are, to some extent, offset by hopes, perhaps overly sanguine, for the domain of the social and the "aesthetic"—a category Kant virtually invented. Even here, however, Kant's hopes were almost outpaced by his forebodings. "We are cultivated," he said, to a remarkable degree; we are civilized "perhaps to excess." But as for being moralized, "much is lacking."[52]

The challenge for moral philosophy, as Kant sees it, is not so much a facile skepticism (as with some recent interpreters) as a despair grounded in the judgments of esteem and contempt from which the moral impulse of the soul also arises. Kant's conception of human dignity, it could be said, is a translation and transformation of biblical morality especially suited to liberal-democratic times (although Kant himself would not so qualify matters), or, alternatively, to times in which politics in an older sense takes the form of an assertion of men's right to constitutional self-government. Human dignity, for Kant, is grounded in a combination of self-exaltation and abasement, honor, and humility. In the tension this provokes lies one source of the extraordinary power and variability of Kant's influence. Man, in Kant's view, must justify creation itself—a task that earlier thinkers did not deem possible or necessary. The result is a new emphasis on history, or mankind as collective subject—an understanding that paved the way for the political disasters of the twentieth century.

That Kant did not himself go down this road stems in no small measure from his rejection, on moral grounds, of a humanity conceptualized wholly historically. Against the relativity of values that otherwise threatens to absorb all human doings, Kant posits moral personality, or the capacity of the individual to merit punishment and reward, as the one quality that renders us (or any other finite being) nonfungible. Where punishment (and reward) are concerned, no one can rightly take another's place.[53]

Kant's association of the idea of dignity (or incomparable worth) with individual responsibility has obvious moral and political appeal, as anyone who has railed against "group guilt" can readily perceive. Kant's association of dignity with the capacity to have actions imputed to one also has certain conceptual advantages—especially given the collapse, under the auspices of modern natural science, of traditional philosophic and religious claims to knowledge of the human good. In the absence of such claims, the irreplaceability of the deserving subject is all that stands between us and a world in which anything can have a price and nothing has intrinsic value—a universe, as Kant suggests, that thoughtful human beings would not choose to enter upon anew.

Can moral personality (so understood) bear the philosophic and existential weight that Kant places on it? Perhaps. Certainly the notion of desert on which it rests strikes a deep and powerful chord. Kant speaks to a common, prescientific sense of justice and nobility that an earlier liberalism was wont to slight. Human dignity finds immediate witness in our most ordinary experiences of moral indignation, be it directed inward (as conscience) or outward (as punitive anger toward others). That the freedom we attribute to the object of our anger makes it, willy-nilly, into an object of respect is one jarring note in an account otherwise easy to accommodate to what he called the "ordinary moral understanding."[54]

Whatever one finally makes of this fact, there is surely something attractive—even bracing—in his honorable defense of democratic virtue. Dignity, for Kant, is necessarily equal as well as measureless. We transcend the realm of price by virtue of our shared capacity to obey the law of which we are ourselves the author. At a time in which material progress (or, as we now say, change) is likely to accelerate precipitously, we could do worse than ponder the assertion on which Kant pegged his own political hopes: "No being endowed with freedom is satisfied with the enjoyment of life's comforts that are apportioned to him by another. . . . What matters is rather the principle according to which he provides it for himself."[55]

Notes

1. Cf. the use, now mainly archaic, of "worthy" as a synonym for "dignitary."

2. The classic study is Ernst H. Kantorowicz, *The King's Two Bodies: A Study in Medieval Political Theology* (Princeton: Princeton University Press, 1957).

3. As has often been noted, Kant's moral views and his understanding of human dignity in particular draw partly on the Stoic natural law tradition. For perhaps his earliest thematic discussion of Stoic doctrines concerning freedom and necessity (a rehearsal, to a remarkable degree, of his later treatment of the "third antinomy"), see his *Nova Delucidatio* (1756), in Kant, *Werke,* Akademie Edition (Berlin: Walter de Gruyter, 1914–), vol. 2; translated in Kant, *Theoretical Philosophy, 1755–1770* [The Cambridge Edition of the Works of Immanuel Kant] (Cambridge: Cambridge University Press, 1992). (All citations of Kant's works refer, first, to the German Akademie edition, followed, after a semicolon, by citation of an English translation where available. Translations provided in the text are my own.) Kant's emphasis on "personality," a term reserved in medieval times largely for the "three persons" of the Trinity, also borrows, both terminologically and conceptually, from Roman law. (On medieval conceptions of the "person," see *The Catholic Encyclopedia.* See also Robert P. Kraynak, chapter 3 in this volume.)

4. Kant's notion of freedom as autonomy (or self-legislation, as distinguished from *autarky* [or self-rule]) decisively distinguishes his thought from that of the Stoics, for whom self-rule is mediated by reason, which they understand to be an active principle, accessible to theoretical knowledge, that permeates the universe— an understanding of reason that Kant explicitly rejects. Reason, for Kant, is associated with the self and its powers of origination (i.e., "spontaneitas"), rather than, as with the Stoics, contemplative participation in an order beyond the self.

5. Kant, *Gesammelte Schriften,* XX 44.

6. For a different interpretation, see Cummiskey, *Kantian Consequentialism,* 75–80.

7. *Metaphysics of Morals,* VI 223; trans. Mary Gregor (Cambridge: Cambridge University Press, 1991), 50.

8. *Critique of Practical Reason,* V 31; trans. Lewis White Beck (Indianapolis: Bobbs-Merrill, 1956), 31. See also Juvenal, *Satire* vi. 223: "This is my will, this is my command; my will is reason enough." The context, strangely enough, is the (wrongful) condemnation (by a shrewish mistress) of a slave whose humanity is also put in question. The entire passage, which epitomizes justice gone awry, should be compared to Juvenal's later praise of the incorruptible witness—a passage Kant cites in the same work as an exemplar of moral instruction (*Satires* 8.79–84; quoted by Kant [V 159; 163]). (For another instance of Kant's willingness to appropriate satire to his own use, see the opening of *Perpetual Peace.*)

9. All necessary propositions, as Kant elsewhere argues, are true by virtue of their *a priority* or origin in reason, as distinguished from empirical perception. This claim is intended, in part, as a response to Humean skepticism.

10. VI 434–35; 230.

11. For helpful discussions of Kant's argument, see Thomas E. Hill, Jr., *Dignity and Practical Reason in Kant's Moral Theory* (Ithaca: Cornell University Press, 1992), 47–50; and David Cummiskey, *Kant's Consequentialism* (New York: Oxford University Press, 1996), 127–31.

12. IV 434–35; 40–41.

13. One can also understand the "pricelessness" of personality as flowing from the fact that moral desert is not transferable. No person can assume another's guilt. See, in this regard, Kant's *Lectures on Ethics* (Vigilantius), XXVII 594; *Lectures on Ethics* (The Cambridge Edition of Kant's Works [Cambridge: Cambridge University Press, 1997]), 342. The implications for orthodox notions of Christ's redemption go without saying.

14. V 162; 166.

15. Cf. Kraynak, chapter 3 in this volume. To the extent that one identifies dignity with immortality simply, it becomes difficult to distinguish different degrees of dignity (can some creatures be more immortal than others?).

16. In the *Lectures on Ethics* (transcribed by Vigilantius), Kant defines "humanity" as follows: "To make a rule for oneself presupposes that we set our intelligible self, i.e., humanity in our own person, over against our sensible being, i.e., man in our own person, and thus contrast man as the agent with the law-giving party.... *Humanity is the aforementioned noumenon, and thus thought of as pure intelligence in regard to the capacity for freedom and accountability implanted in man. Man, on the other hand, is humanity in appearance, and thus subordinated to humanity as genus*" (emphasis added) (XXVII 579; 330). Man, for Kant, is, in this peculiar sense, a species being.

17. *Grounding of the Metaphysics of Morals*, IV 429; 36.

18. *Metaphysics of Morals*, VI 422–23; 219.

19. *Metaphysics of Morals*, VI 429; 226.

20. The individual who lies remains, as it were, empirically a man, but internally forfeits his connection with the noumenal. Hence, Kant's claim that a liar "throws away his dignity."

21. *Metaphysics of Morals*, VI 435; 230–31.

22. Cf. Jean-François Lyotard, *The Differend: Phrases in Dispute*, trans. Georges Van Den Abbeele (Minneapolis: University of Minnesota Press, 1983), 161–81. Lyotard rightly stresses the paradoxically transpositional (or "passage-like") character of this response, especially in light of Kant's underlying dualism. His reading fails to acknowledge, however, the distinction on which Kant himself insists in the *Critique of Judgment* between the "noble" (or genuinely moral) and

the "enthusiastic" (or merely aesthetic) sublime, a distinction that leaves the wall between reason and feeling intact (V 272). To be sure, at least one of Kant's later works assigns enthusiasm a somewhat higher status. The *Anthropology*, for example, describes enthusiasm as the "cause" of affect (not, as he had earlier claimed, affect itself), and, as such, compatible with "reason holding the reins," as in political or spiritual addresses that "enliven" the people's will—an example especially revealing for present purposes. (For a fuller treatment of this issue, see Susan M. Shell, *The Embodiment of Reason: Kant on Spirit, Generation and Community* [Chicago: University of Chicago Press, 1996], 273 and n. 63.)

23. See Alex Kaufman, *Welfare in the Kantian State* (London: Oxford University Press, 1999), for a helpful treatment of the historical setting.

24. As in *"Abbruch."*

25. See Lincoln's "Address at the Wisconsin State Fair, 1859," in *The Political Thought of Abraham Lincoln,* ed. Richard N. Current (Indianapolis: Bobbs-Merrill, 1967), 124–36.

26. Cf. Thomas Aquinas, *Summa Theologica,* 2a2ae.64.3. For Kant retributive justice honors the criminal's human dignity—a dignity that, for Aquinas, the criminal specifically forfeits.

27. This general consideration allows us to make better sense of Kant's notorious distinction between policies that a people "could" and "could not" consent to. Basically, Kant's view seems to be that a policy contrary to right is permissible in the short run if it can be interpreted by the people as a temporary concession to circumstances (on the theory that [almost] anything is better than a reversion to the state of nature). An unambiguous public declaration that human beings, as such, have no rights, on the other hand, would constitute an overturning of justice itself. In the *Conflict of the Faculties,* Kant notes that no ruler has ever made such a pronouncement or ever will, out of foreknowledge that such a declaration would provoke the people to rise up in fury against him (VII 87n.; 156n.). For a similar discussion of the issue of inherited titles, see *Metaphysics of Morals,* VI 329; 138–39.

28. See the note appended to a remark "important," as Kant puts it, "to anthropology": "Why has a ruler never dared freely to declare that he recognizes no right of the people against him; that his people owe their happiness solely to the *beneficence* of a government that confers it on them, and that all presumption of the subject to a right opposed to the government . . . is absurd and even punishable? The reason is that such public declaration would rouse all subjects against him; although as docile sheep, led by a benevolent and sensible master, well-fed and powerfully protected, they would have nothing wanting in their welfare about which to complain" (*Conflict of the Faculties,* VII 86n.–87n.; 155n.–157n.).

29. See Leo Strauss, "Preface," *Spinoza's Critique of Religion* (New York: Schocken, 1965), 2.

30. *Idea for a Universal History from a Cosmopolitan Standpoint* (VIII 18); in Kant, *Political Writings*, 2nd ed., trans. Hans Reiss (Cambridge: Cambridge University Press, 1991), 42.

31. *Critique of Judgment*, V 435; trans. Werner Pluhar (Indianapolis: Hackett, 1987), 322–23.

32. *Tauglichkeit*, as Kant himself points out, is cognate with *Tügend* (virtue).

33. *Critique of Judgment*, V 431; 319.

34. *Critique of Judgment*, V 432, 434–36; 320, 322–23.

35. See *Perpetual Peace*, "First Supplement: On the Guarantee of a Perpetual Peace." Most standard English translations render Kant's "für ["for"]" inaccurately as "by."

36. Cf. *Idea for a Universal History*, thesis 6.

37. See *Perpetual Peace*, second appendix; for an extended discussion, see Susan M. Shell, "Bowling Alone: On the Saving Power of Kant's 'Perpetual Peace,'" *Idealistic Studies* (Spring 1996): 53–73; and "Cannibals All: The Grave Wit of Kant's 'Perpetual Peace,'" in Samuel Weber and Hent de Vries, eds., *Violence, Identity and Self-Determination* (Stanford: Stanford University Press, 1997), 150–61.

38. *Conflict of the Faculties*, VII 89; trans. Mary Gregor (New York: Abaris, 1979), 161.

39. By "sympathy" here, Kant does not mean pathological "good-heartedness," but something closer to the Stoic ideal of *sympatheia*, or the intimate connection between God and humans by virtue of which all the wise and virtuous are friends (see "Stoicism," in *Encyclopaedia Britannica* [11th ed.]). Cf. *Metaphysics of Morals*, VI 456–57.

40. See pp. 59–60 above.

41. *Conflict of the Faculties*, VII 89; 161.

42. See *Conflict of the Faculties*, VII 82; 147.

43. Human reason, as he asserts at the conclusion of the *Groundwork*, cannot grasp the "practical unconditioned necessity of the moral imperative" and, indeed cannot be blamed for failing to do so, for this would be to explain that necessity in terms of a condition (i.e., some underlying interest), in which case it would cease to be moral. All we can "fairly ask" philosophy, which "strives in its principles to reach the very limit of human reason," to do is grasp the "inconceivability" of that necessity—the inconceivability, that is to say, of freedom's possibility (IV 424; 62).

44. Compare the argument of Rousseau's "Savoyard Vicar" in *Emile*.

45. Compare Kant's critique of an "überschwenglich" (or "high-flying") understanding of moral virtue as consisting in "so-called noble or supermeritorious actions," an understanding that "runs up into empty wishes and longings for unattainable perfection" at the expense of "common and everyday responsibility." A great, selfless, and sympathetic disposition toward humanity is to be prized. Still, "one need only reflect a little to find an indebtedness which he has in some way

incurred to the human race (even if it be only that, by the inequality of men under the civil constitution, he enjoys advantages on account of which others must be lacking to just that extent)," in order that the self-loving image of merit not supplant "the thought of duty" (*Critique of Practical Reason* V 155–56 [and note]; 158–59 [and note]). Greatness of soul in something like the classical sense is specifically discounted as dependent, at least indirectly, on undeserved helps, as well as for its self-complacent elevation of merit over duty. As Kant asserts: "Respect for the law, and not any pretension to inner greatness of mind (*Großmuth*) or noble and meritorious way of thinking . . . exercises the greatest force on the mind (*Gemüth*) of the spectator."

46. *Groundwork of the Metaphysics of Morals*, IV 393; 7.

47. Cf. Leo Strauss, *Liberalism Ancient and Modern* (New York: Basic Books, 1968), 22, who says, apropos of both Rousseau and Kant: "The only thing which can be held to be unqualifiedly good is not the contemplation of the eternal, not the cultivation of the mind, to say nothing of good breeding, but a good intention, and of good intentions everyone is as capable as everyone else, wholly independently of education. Accordingly, the uneducated could even appear to have an advantage over the educated: the voice of nature or the moral law speaks in them perhaps more clearly and more decidedly than in the sophisticated who may have sophisticated away their conscience." In fairness to Kant, it must be said that the problem of (moral) education was the overriding theme of his professional life. (See, for example, his letter to Marcus Herz [April 1778] [X 230–32].)

48. Greatness of soul, for Kant, is replaced by or merges with conscientious striving or willingness to make an effort. Compare John Rawls, who treats such willingness as "arbitrary from a moral point of view," i.e., as an asset as undeserved as are all other natural gifts. (See *A Theory of Justice* [Cambridge: Harvard University Press, 1971], 104, 312.)

49. *Metaphysics of Morals*, VI 380; 186, VI 429–30; 225–26. Kant's two examples of such "inner lying" are: (1) falsely professing belief in a "future judge of the world" in case he should exist, and (2) (in one who genuinely believes) flattering oneself that one reveres the law, when one's actual incentive is fear of punishment—forms of hypocrisy to which, one could add, a skeptical atheism and a dogmatic Christianity are especially prone. Kant's own problem lies in keeping "hope in the future" to which morality, on his account, gives rise, from becoming (or appearing in the guise of) its condition. See in this regard his discussion of the honest or well-meaning atheist in the *Critique of Judgment:* "How will he judge his own inner destination to a purpose (*Zweckbestimmung*) through the law? . . . Deceit, violence, and envy will always be rife around him, even though he himself is honest, peaceable, and benevolent. . . . No matter how worthy of happiness [he or others] may be, nature . . . will subject them all to all the evils [to which other animals are subject] . . . And they will stay subject to these evils always, until one vast tomb engulfs

them one and all (honest or not, that makes no difference here) and hurls them, who managed to believe they were the final purpose of creation, back into the abyss of the purposeless chaos of matter from which they were taken." So, Kant adds, "the well-meaning person would have to give up as impossible the purpose that he, following the moral law, had and had to have before his eyes." Such a person must therefore assume (*annehmen*) the existence of a moral author of the world, in order to avoid damage (*Abbruch*) to his own moral attitude (*moralische Gesinnung*) (V 452–53; 342) (emphasis added).

50. In his late *Announcement of a Near Conclusion of a Treaty of Eternal Peace in Philosophy*, Kant calls "lying" the one "foul spot" that marks the human race (IX 422; trans. in Peter Fenves, *Raising the Tone of Philosophy* [Baltimore: Johns Hopkins University Press, 1993], 93).

51. *Critique of Judgment*, V 434n.; 121n. Compare John Rawls's definition of the "good man" and a "person's good," in terms of the adoption of a "rational life plan" ("rational" being understood in essentially formal terms): "Imagine someone [fanciful] whose only pleasure is to count blades of grass. . . . If we allow that his nature is to enjoy this activity and not to enjoy any other, and there is no feasible way to alter his condition, then . . . a rational plan for him will center on this activity" (*A Theory of Justice*, 432).

52. *Idea for a Universal History*, thesis 7.

53. Cf. *Religion within the Limits of Reason Alone*: radical evil is the "most *personal* of all liabilities," which "only the culprit, not the innocent, can bear." It is the "old Adam," on this view, rather than Jesus Christ, who bears the burden of redemptive sacrifice. See VI: 74–76; trans. George di Giovanni in Kant, *Religion and Rational Theology* (Cambridge, Cambridge University Press, 1996), 114–15.

54. Cf. n. 27.

55. *Conflict of the Faculties*, VII 87n.; 157n.

CHAPTER THREE

"Made in the Image of God": The Christian View of Human Dignity and Political Order

ROBERT P. KRAYNAK

Among the great philosophies and religions of the world, Christianity may be said to make the loftiest claims on behalf of human dignity. In contrast to pagan philosophers such as Aristotle, who pointedly says that "man is not the best thing in the universe" because the heavenly bodies are more perfect (*Ethics,* 1141a21), Christianity builds upon the biblical view that man is made in "the image and likeness of God" and stands at the peak of creation. Judaism and Islam, of course, also exalt humanity above other creatures and see the divine image in man. But Christianity goes beyond the other monotheistic religions in holding as its central article of faith the Incarnation: the belief that God became man in the person of Jesus Christ. As both the Son of God and the Son of Man, Christ lowered the divine nature to assume a human form but in so doing raised human nature by offering the hope of salvation to fallen or sinful human beings. In this spirit, Christianity teaches charity or love for all mankind, from the highest to the lowest individuals in worldly terms; even the humblest may be exalted. Through these fundamental teachings, Christianity makes a powerful statement about the dignity of man.

While the claims of Christianity on behalf of human dignity are undeniable, the precise meaning of those claims as well as their implications for politics are not always clear; understanding them requires theological interpretation and practical judgment. In the contemporary world, the Christian view of human dignity is most often understood in terms of the "human person" and the rights of persons to recognition, respect, and suitable standards of material well-being. Included in this imperative is a conception of social justice that requires democratic norms of equality and democratic political institutions. The significance of this interpretation lies in linking the Christian view of human dignity with human rights and a specific political order—namely, democracy (either the liberal democracy supported by most contemporary Christians or the socialist democracy preferred by liberation theologians).

Despite the broad consensus today among Christians about the democratic implications of human dignity, one should not forget that this interpretation is fairly new and is by no means the only or the best interpretation. It should be recognized as the modern understanding of human dignity, which had to be established against the ancient (patristic and medieval) understandings. One indication of the relative novelty of the current view is that neither the New Testament nor the greatest theologians and church leaders of the Christian tradition promoted democracy as the best political order or spoke in the language of human rights. Indeed, the Christian tradition throughout most of its two-thousand-year history understood human dignity and the political order in ways that were more hierarchical and corporate than liberal and democratic. How do we account for this fact? Why did the traditional spokesmen for Christianity not conceive of human dignity in the democratic terms that seem so self-evident today? Was the older view a distortion of Christianity, or does it contain important insights that we moderns have forgotten or are ashamed to admit?

In attempting to answer these questions, I shall first inquire into the biblical meaning of human dignity, which is largely a matter of interpreting passages referring to the image of God in man. My principal claim is that the Bible uses the term "image of God" to describe the high point in the created hierarchy of beings without specifying precisely what qualities or attributes justify that ranking. While man's original possession of immortality may be the attribute closest to God, it has been obscured or lost and implies the need for divine redemption rather than political claims of democratic equality or human rights.

After discussing the Bible, I will turn to the early church and medieval theologians in order to show that they also conceive of dignity as a type of rank in the created hierarchy; but they add the insight of Greek philosophy that the source of human dignity is the possession of a rational soul. Yet, even this addition, which includes the notion of free will, does not contain an imperative for democracy or rights because the rational soul is primarily directed toward knowing and loving the first cause of its being, namely, God, which is a spiritual rather than a political imperative. Finally, I will examine the modern Christian understanding of human dignity and will argue that it develops the divine image in terms of Kantian philosophy: Dignity comes to mean the infinite worth of the human person who claims respect as a right. My aim is to show that the modern view is the least persuasive of the three because it treats human dignity as an absolute right rather than as a matter of degree in a hierarchy of perfection, producing a view of Christian faith that is overly political and that diminishes the spiritual value of subordinating the human personality to a higher order of being. The true Christian view of human dignity, I hope to show, is more compatible with hierarchy than with democracy, though it permits an accommodation with modern democracy for prudential reasons.

The Biblical View of Human Dignity

In reflecting on the Christian view of human dignity, scholars commonly begin with the biblical references to the *Imago Dei*—to the image of God in man. For example, Reinhold Niebuhr argues in *The Nature and Destiny of Man* that the human quality most reflective of the divine nature is "self-transcendence": the capacity to rise above our natural selves and freely construct a world of higher meanings.[1] A different formulation is offered by Eric Voegelin, who says that the "Christian notion of 'human dignity' is the common divinity in all men" or "the equal spiritual dignity of all men," which contrasts with the pagan philosophers' "inclination to treat non-philosophical man as an inferior brand and even to compare him to animals."[2] Another striking statement comes from Pope John Paul II: "God has imprinted His own image and likeness on man, conferring upon him an incomparable dignity . . . beyond the rights which man acquires by his own work, there exist rights which do not correspond to any work he performs, but which flow from his essential dignity as a person."[3] And, in a surprising parallel, one can find in *The Rights of Man* by Tom Paine the claim that the "divine principle of the equal rights of man . . . has its origin from the Maker of man"; it is found in the biblical "account of creation, [where] 'God said, Let us make man in our own image' . . . [which] shows that the equality of man, so far from being a modern doctrine, is the oldest upon record."[4] This last statement, of course, is an expression of the fundamental American article of faith that all human beings have equal rights because everyone is a child of God.[5]

As these diverse figures attest, the biblical view of the *Imago Dei* is a powerful claim, from which important inferences about human nature, morality, and politics have been drawn. Yet, if one actually examines the Bible carefully, one is struck by how difficult it is to make such inferences. There are only a few explicit references to the *Imago Dei* in both the Old and New Testaments, and they are ambiguous about what precisely constitutes the divine image in man: Is it reason, language, free will, soul, a physical trait (such as upright posture), immortality, or capacities for love, holiness, and justice? Moreover, the Bible is very spare in drawing moral and political implications from this image. A brief survey of the relevant passages will indicate the power and elusiveness of the biblical *Imago Dei*.

Three references appear in Genesis. The first and most famous occurs in the account of creation: "Then God said, 'Let us make man in our image (*tzelem*), after our likeness (*demuth*); and let them have dominion over the fish of the sea, and over the birds of the air, and over the cattle, and over all the earth, and over every creeping thing that creeps upon the earth.' So God created man in his own image, in the image of God he created him, male and female he created them" (Gen. 1:26–27). A second passage draws a parallel between God's creation and Adam's procreation: "This is the book of the generation of Adam. When God created man, he made him in the likeness of God. Male and female he created them, and he blessed them and named them Man (*adam*) when they were created. When Adam had lived a hundred and thirty years, he became the father of a son in his own likeness, after his image, and named him Seth" (Gen. 5:1–3). A third passage occurs in the story of the Flood after the waters receded; God blesses Noah and his family using the language of Genesis to teach the value of human life: "Be fruitful and multiply, and fill the earth. The fear and the dread of you shall be upon every beast of the earth . . . For your lifeblood I will surely require a reckoning . . . Whoever sheds the blood of man, by man shall his blood be shed; for God made man in his own image" (Gen. 9:5–7).

These three passages are the only references in Genesis (and indeed in the entire Hebrew Bible) to the *Imago Dei* and are therefore the primary basis for understanding the biblical conception of human dignity. They show that God has created the natural world as a hierarchy with the human species at the top, possessing a special right of dominion over the lower species. But this dominion is not unlimited or arbitrary. In the first grant of dominion, man is commanded to subdue the birds, fish, and cattle but his food is restricted to plants—a sort of primitive dietary law of vegetarianism (Gen. 1:29–30). When Adam and Eve are created in the Garden, they are further restricted by the prohibition not to eat of the tree of the knowledge of good and evil, lest they die. After they disobey, whatever human dignity they previously possessed is henceforth combined with depravity and with mortality; but their dignity is not entirely lost. In fact, in the story of Noah, the grant of dominion is renewed and the image of God reaffirmed. According to the second grant of dominion to Noah, the primitive vegetarianism is expanded to include the flesh of animals as food, but the blood must be drained (Gen. 9:4). In addition, man is elevated by the respect that must be shown to human life. This demand almost resembles a right to life, except that it includes the death penalty for taking a life, which seems to imply, as the scholar Cassuto notes, that a "murderer has . . . erased the divine likeness from himself by his act of murder."[6]

We may thus infer that the divine image in man is a sign of special favor from God—a comparative rank entitling man to limited dominion over creatures that may be seen as a mirror of God's total dominion over all creation. Yet, the divine image is something that can be compromised or partially lost, either by the whole human species or by individuals who commit immoral acts such as murder. In addition to stressing dominion over the earth, these passages from Genesis emphasize procreation, as if procreation were also a quality reflective of God. Sometimes the Bible seems to be saying that God's ability to create is mirrored in man's ability to procreate; hence the reference to sexual differentiation of male and female as part of the divine image and the blessing or command to "be fruitful and multiply." Although the ability to procreate enables man to make children in his image—just as God made Adam in his image, so Adam makes Seth in his image—one cannot be sure if this is the basis of human dignity. For the lower animals also procreate "according to their kinds" and are blessed or commanded to "be fruitful and multiply" in the same language as man (Gen. 1:22). Perhaps the Bible is suggesting that procreation with the conscious intention of dominion over the earth is the divine image in man (which may explain why environmentalists and population control experts are troubled by Genesis).

The difficulty is that these three passages in Genesis give us a tantalizing glimpse into human dignity by referring to the divine image in man without precisely defining its qualities and conditions. The divine image seems to refer primarily to man's rank in the created hierarchy and to grants of restricted dominion over other creatures. Morally, it seems to confer special worth to human life and to procreation through male-female sexual differentiation, although the lifeblood and procreation of other animals also receives certain blessings (as if they too shared to some extent in the divine image and deserve a certain respect, diminishing the absolute uniqueness of man and suggesting limits on environmental usage).[7]

If this is true, however, what remains of the special dignity of man? The only answer that makes sense to me is that the lifeblood and procreation which man admittedly shares with other animals has a deeper meaning for the human species: It is a pale reflection of something that man alone possessed before the Fall, namely, immortal life. The implication is that immortality is the lost image of God in man—a suggestion supported not only by the account of the Fall, which is primarily about the loss of immortality, but also by the longevity of Adam and the early patriarchs, who lived up to 900 years, as a kind of afterglow of immortality, which God finally ended by arbitrarily setting the limit to human life at 120 years (Gen. 6:3). As compensation for the limited life span of mortal individuals, the surrogate immortality that Adam found in his son Seth continues through the procreation of families and tribes that endure for generations, as Abram soon learns when God makes him Abraham, the father of his people. Man's dignity, in the sense of original immortality or surrogate immortality (through procreation and longevity), is therefore not absolute but comparative: It is the highest degree of perfection in the created hierarchy.

After the rich and suggestive passages of Genesis, the only other passages in the Old Testament that directly address the dignity of man are those in Psalm 8, Wisdom 2:23–24, and Ecclesiasticus 17:1–12. Although Psalm 8 does not include the phrase "image of God," it uses the unmistakable language of Genesis to describe man's place in the universe. The psalmist expresses his wonder that God created the moon and the stars in the heavens and yet, in the vast universe, cares above all for the human creature: "What is man that thou art mindful of him? . . . Yet thou hast made him a little less than God [or a little less than the angels or divine beings; in Hebrew *elohim*] and dost crown him with glory and honor. Thou hast given him dominion over the works of thy hands . . . [over] sheep and oxen, and also the birds of the air and the fish of the sea" (8:4–8). The lines of this psalm are a classic example of biblical minimalism: Man's dignity—his glory and honor—is expressed with loving wonder, and man's dominion over the lower animals is bluntly asserted. But no reasons are given for God's favor. The selection of the human species for special care and dominion is comparable in its mystery to the special selection of Israel from among the myriad tribes and nations, a reflection of the inscrutable will of YHWH who Is What He Is without giving reasons.

By contrast, the books of Wisdom and Ecclesiasticus (which are not included in the canonical Hebrew Bible but are part of the Old Testament in most Christian Bibles) supply reasons for man's dignity, reflecting perhaps their later composition when Greek philosophical influences encouraged rational explanations. According to Wisdom 2:23–24, "For God created man for incorruption, and made him *in the image of his own eternity*, but through the devil's envy death entered the world" (emphasis added). Here is the most explicit identification of the divine image in man with the specific attribute of incorruption or immortality, either of soul or body or both together. The passages from Ecclesiasticus 17:1–12 follow the same pattern of defining the image of God in terms of attributes: "The Lord created man out of earth, and turned him back to it again. He gave to men few days, a limited time, but granted them authority over things upon the earth. He endowed them with *strength like his own, and made them in his own image*. He

placed the fear of them in all living beings and granted them dominion over beasts and birds. He made for them tongue and eyes; he gave
them ears and *a mind for thinking. He filled them with knowledge and
understanding* and showed them good and evil . . . He bestowed knowledge upon them, and allotted to them the law of life . . . [and an] eternal
covenant" (emphasis added). In this passage, the echoes of Genesis are
evident in the references to human dominion over creatures, but the
emphasis on attributes such as Godlike strength (a puzzling notion) and
reason or understanding (through the senses, language, and heart) give
a more precise elaboration of the *Imago Dei*.

Yet, it is not clear if any of these attributes are as important as the
simple fact of God's election of man for special care and the election
of Israel for a special "eternal" covenant. In this sense, the *Imago Dei*—
as God's mysterious selection of certain beings for divine favors and his
promise never to abandon them—is the premise of the entire Old
Testament, which may explain why it appears prominently in Genesis
up to the first covenant (with Noah) and then drops out of sight. The
references in the wisdom literature that equate the image of God with
lost immortality and rationality are helpful but not definitive for interpreting Genesis.

A further complication is that the books of Exodus, Leviticus, and
the latter Hebrew prophets avoid direct references to the *Imago Dei* of
Genesis, yet they clearly compare man with God in the capacity for
holiness (*kadosh*). The command "You shall be holy, for I am holy" (Lev.
11:45) is forcefully stated as the reason for obeying the divine law. The
implication seems to be that God no longer draws man toward divinity
through the surrogate immortality of the family of Abraham but through
the divine law, revealed to Moses, which requires holiness. Indeed, the
express purpose of the Mosaic law is to make a "holy nation" (Exod.
19:6) through a myriad of commands that require the utmost devotion.
To be "holy" in this sense has many connotations that are hard to define
precisely. In a formal and almost tautological sense, holiness means
being set apart from the profane. But it also implies separation from the
profane in specific ways—by superior purity in sexual and dietary matters, by transcendence of the mundane through the mysterious presence
of the invisible God, and by a high degree of righteousness in the exe-
cution of justice and social responsibilities. The divine image in man
found almost exclusively in the book of Genesis is thus superseded but

not abolished by the imitation of God's holiness in observing the divine law—making people more Godlike in their purity, transcendence, and righteousness. Perhaps the Hebrew Bible is saying that lost image of God from Genesis (the lost immortality of Adam and Eve) may be recovered through the gifts of family and law—partly by continuing forever the extended family of Abraham but also and above all by keeping the eternal covenant and obeying the Law of Moses, which makes people holy like the Holy One of Israel.[8]

It is not until we arrive at the New Testament that the original language of Genesis about the *Imago Dei* reappears in the Bible. Here, we find about a dozen references to the image, likeness, figure, and form of God as well as a variety of loose references to similar notions such as the children of God, the sons of God, and "partakers of the divine nature." Some of these terms are reserved especially for Jesus Christ, who is called "the image (*eikon*) of the invisible God, the first-born of all creation" (Col. 1:15; 2 Cor. 4:4) and "the figure (*character*) of His substance" (Heb. 1:3). These descriptions are clearly intended to connect the *Imago Dei* of Genesis with the central article of the Christian faith—the Incarnation, in which the invisible God becomes a visible man in Jesus Christ. As Paul says of Christ, "though he was in the form of God, he did not count equality with God a thing to be grasped, but emptied himself, taking the form of a servant, being born in the likeness of men" (Phil. 2:5–7; Heb. 2:5–18).

The point of using the language of image and likeness from Genesis to explain the birth of Christ may be inferred from Paul's theology: While God originally created man in the divine image, that image has been obscured or lost; hence, it needs to be restored by Christ, who is the real image of God. Unlike the foolish pagans, who "exchange the glory of the immortal God for images resembling mortal men or birds or animals or reptiles" (Rom. 1:20–23), Christians see the real image of God in the immortal man, Jesus Christ. Christ combines in his person the image of God (immortality) and the likeness of fallen men (mortality) and therefore is able to restore the lost image of God to man (to restore lost immortality).

Although Paul tends to reserve the *Imago Dei* for Christ, he also applies it in a different manner to ordinary mortals. In one of his most controversial statements, he sees a further, if dimmer, reflection of the image of God in men—specifically, in males as the head of the household: "The head of every man is Christ, the head of a woman is her husband, and the head of Christ is God . . . [hence] a man ought not to cover his head, since he is the image and glory of God; but the woman is the glory of man . . . [and] ought to have a veil on her head" (1 Cor. 11:3–16). The reason Paul gives is that "man was not made from woman, but woman from man," meaning that Eve was created from Adam's rib; but he cautions that man's authority over woman is also a kind of reciprocity, for "man is now born of woman; and all things are from God." What is significant about Paul's statement is that he uses the image of God as it was used in the Old Testament: to establish a hierarchy according to the order of divine creation. Here, the hierarchy extends from God to Christ to man to woman and is justified not in terms of natural superiority based on some preferred attributes but on the supernatural, and ultimately mysterious, creation of God. Nevertheless, Paul indicates that the created order may in some sense be thought of as "natural" and even ought to be reflected in social conventions, such as women covering their heads as a sign of modesty.[9] A kind of continuum thereby emerges from created hierarchies to natural hierarchies to social hierarchies.

Herein lies the fundamental difference between the biblical and the contemporary understanding of human dignity. In the biblical view, dignity is hierarchical and comparative; in the modern, it is democratic and absolute. The Bible (both Old and New Testaments) promotes hierarchies because it understands reality in terms of the "image of God," which is a type of reflected glory—a reflection of something more perfect. Hence, dignity exists in degrees of perfection rather than in abstractions that are absolutely uniform. Moreover, the dignity or glory possessed by something made in the image of a more perfect being carries moral claims of deference, reciprocal obligation, and duty rather than equality, freedom, and rights. Christ is bound to the dominion of the Father and Creator; man is bound to the dominion of Christ; woman is bound to the dominion of man; and, reciprocally, God is bound in love to Christ, Christ to man, man to woman.

Following the logic of reciprocal obligations, there is no contradiction between the statements of the New Testament that require obedience to hierarchies—whether they be divinely created, natural, or conventional—and passages that speak of the spiritual dignity of all human beings. This point needs emphasis because nothing is more con-

fusing for modern Christians than to read passages in the Gospels and
Epistles commanding obedience to the Roman Emperor and acceptance of the patriarchal household and of social inequalities, including
slavery, and then to read other passages asserting that all are one in
Christ and all have a divine spark within them.

For example, we find, on the one side, passages implying that all
people have spiritual dignity and may even become divinized in some
sense—a kind of spiritual democracy. The most well-known passages
are: "There is neither Jew nor Greek, slave nor freeman, male nor
female, for you are all one in Christ" (Gal. 3:28); and through Christ's
"divine power . . . you may . . . become partakers of the divine nature"
(2 Pet. 1:3–4). Yet, in apparent contradiction, we also hear harsh, undemocratic statements such as "Render to Caesar the things that are
Caesar's" (Matt. 22:21); "Let every soul be subject to the governing authorities" (Rom. 13:1; also 1 Pet. 2:13); "Wives, be subject to your hus-
bands, as to the Lord" (Eph. 5:22; also 1 Cor. 11:3, 1 Pet. 3:1); "Slaves, be
obedient to your earthly masters" (Eph. 6:5–7; also Col. 3:18–25, Titus
2:1–10); "I permit not woman to teach or to have authority over men"
(1 Tim. 2:12); and "Go into all the world and preach the Gospel . . .
He who believes and is baptized will be saved; but he who does not
believe will be condemned" (Mark 16:15). Are these statements a denial
of the universal spiritual dignity implied in the previous passages?

The answer, I believe, is that no contradiction exists because the
biblical understanding of dignity is hierarchical: It proclaims the spiritual dignity of every person in some fashion but permits and even
requires different degrees of dignity in the created and natural orders.
The Bible also seems to imply that while dignity in some sense is given
and therefore "inalienable" (as we would say today), it is also something
to be won or lost, merited or forfeited, augmented or diminished. And
it implies that obedience to hierarchical authorities, such as sovereigns
and masters, who are a part of the fallen world and largely conventional
in status, does not violate the dignity of the Christian believer because
real dignity lies in the possession of an immortal soul with a supernatural destiny and in the spiritual freedom of the "innermost self"
(Rom. 7:22).

Some of these points may be inferred from passages which allude
to the divine spark within everyone and to the children of God. When
Peter says (as quoted above) that through Christ we may become

partakers of divinity, he adds the qualification that divinization or exaltation is only attained through virtue: Christ's "divine power has granted to us all things . . . that through these you may escape from the corruption that is in the world from passion, and become partakers of the divine nature. For this very reason make every effort to supplement your faith with virtue, and virtue with knowledge, and knowledge with self-control, and self-control with steadfastness, and steadfastness with godliness, and godliness with brotherly affection, and . . . love" (2 Pet. 1:3–8). The implications of Peter's words are spiritually undemocratic because they link divinization with virtue (moral, intellectual, and spiritual), which cannot be attained by everyone because it requires effort. Peter also says that virtue requires zeal in confirming one's "call and election," a curious mixture of freedom and grace. Partaking in divinity, then, enhances the glory, excellence, or dignity of some but not all, creating a sort of spiritual aristocracy of those who "will be richly provided for . . . [in] the eternal kingdom" (ibid., 1:10–11).

Likewise, when Paul speaks of the sons or children of God, he makes distinctions of rank based on moral and spiritual virtue. The primary distinction, of course, is between those who live by the flesh and those who live by the spirit. Hence, he says, "if you live according to the flesh you will die, but if by the spirit . . . you will live. For all who are led by the Spirit of God are sons of God . . . [and] children of God" (Rom. 8:13–16). But who are they? Paul indicates that they are the few predestined saints: "For the creation waits with eager longing for the revealing of the sons of God . . . [when] the Spirit intercedes for the saints according to the will of God . . . For those whom He foreknew he also predestined to be conformed to the image of his Son . . . [and to be] glorified" (ibid., 8:19, 27–30). In this teaching, Paul simply seems to be restating John's Gospel, "to all who . . . believed in his name, he gave the power to become children of God, who were born not of blood nor of the will of the flesh . . . but of God" (1:12). A more mystical view of the children of God can be found in the Epistle of 1 John (3:1–10), where they are distinguished from the children of the devil by their moral purity and are rewarded with the vision of God and with divinization: "Beloved, we are God's children now; it does not yet appear what we shall be, but you know that when He appears we shall be like Him, for we shall see Him face to face. And everyone who thus hopes in Him purifies himself as He is pure . . . By this it may be seen who are the children of God and who are the children of the devil." This passage is often read as a glimpse of the beatific vision in heaven, where those who are saved by their pure lives—the true children of God—will see God face to face and become like him.

The hierarchical character of spiritual dignity expressed in these passages may be summarized in two general points about biblical Christianity. First, dignity is expressed in the language of image, likeness, form, participation, sonship, and children of God because dignity is a type of reflected glory from a more perfect to a less perfect being. Indeed, this is the very meaning of the word "glory," which is so abundantly used in the New Testament (usually a translation of the Greek *doxa* meaning reputation, honor, glory, and also appearance, seeming, opinion). Glory is the closest word to "dignity" in the New Testament, and it is almost always used to express a hierarchical relation among more or less perfect beings: In the Transfiguration, Christ, Moses, and Elijah "appeared in glory" (Luke 9:30–32); resurrected bodies are "raised in glory" (1 Cor. 15:43); man is the "image and glory of God," and woman is "the glory of man" (1 Cor. 11:7); and in the cosmos "there are celestial bodies and terrestrial bodies; but the glory of the celestial is one, and the glory of the terrestrial is another . . . [every] star differs from star in glory" (1 Cor. 15:40). Thus, there are different glories or degrees of dignity for the whole universe as well as for the Creator and Savior of the universe; and the scale of the hierarchy, while not simply reducible to attributes, is most often measured by degrees of corruptibility and incorruptibility or of mortality and immortality.

The second point to observe is that biblical Christianity seems to distinguish created and natural hierarchies from conventional or social hierarchies. The created and natural hierarchies are upheld as expressions of the divine will, while the conventional hierarchies are upheld as matters of prudence because they inculcate good habits. Thus, the created hierarchy is stated most strongly, extending from the invisible God to his image in the visible Son of God, Christ, to the sons or children of God who through personal effort and election attain virtue. This overlaps to some extent with the natural hierarchy, which includes the image of God in the male head of the household and the female as helpmate and their dominion over the lower species. And both of these overlap to some extent with various accounts of the church hierarchy, which Paul calls the "body of Christ" and compares to the parts of the human body in order to show that the comparative ranking of apostles, prophets, teachers, miracle workers, healers, helpers, administrators, and speakers in tongues are harmoniously ordered (1 Cor. 12:1–13).[10]

In addition to these hierarchies, there is the social and political order, which is largely conventional in character because Christ has distinguished the realm of God from the realm of Caesar. This means that the state (or form of government) and social classes (the distribution of wealth, honor, power) are not precisely determined by created or natural hierarchies. Hence, the question of the best political regime is left unanswered in the New Testament. Instead, it states that the established state and social classes, including the unequal distribution of power and wealth, are to be obeyed for prudential reasons. As Peter says, "Be subject for the Lord's sake to every human institution," which means that Christian citizens should accept the authority of the Roman Emperor and Christian slaves should accept the authority of their masters not as natural superiors but "for the Lord's sake"—because God willed these institutions as restraints on sinful human nature and to teach lessons of reciprocal obligation between master and servant and between rich and poor ("As for the rich of this world, charge them not to be haughty . . . [but] to be rich in good deeds, liberal and generous" [1 Tim. 6:17–19]). The strangeness of this teaching is that it requires accepting conventions as mere conventions, even while recognizing that the poor and the powerless are closer to God in their humility and charity.[11]

In the last analysis, the New Testament teaches the difficult message of obedience to created, natural, and conventional hierarchies because the dignity of every person is ultimately a matter of inner, spiritual freedom that is radically independent of the social-political order and may even be deepened by external servitude rather than by grants of external freedom. In other words, the Christian freedom spoken of in the New Testament and boldly proclaimed by Paul—"For freedom, Christ has set us free . . . do not submit to a yoke of slavery" (Gal. 5:1)—is not a reference to what we today call rights or to the struggle against oppression or even to emancipation from the social institution of slavery. As Orlando Patterson rightly argues in *Freedom and the Making of Western Culture,* Paul is speaking of "spiritual freedom"—meaning the liberation of the soul from sin through the agency of personal struggle against temptation and the saving grace of Jesus Christ. Patterson is undoubtedly correct in arguing that Paul took from the Roman institutions of his day the rhetoric of slavery, emancipation, and redemption ("you are not your own . . . you were bought with a price" [1 Cor. 6:19]). But Patterson is misleading in suggesting that Paul sees manumission as the logical culmination of Christian freedom or that "medieval and later Christianity morally sanctioned servitude, but this charge cannot be laid on Paul."[12] Paul's position is that slavery to sin is worse than slavery to another man, which makes the latter a question of prudence that in most cases counsels acceptance of external servitude.

Hence, in the Epistle to Philemon, Paul commands a fugitive slave, Onesimus, to return to his master, Philemon, and the master to receive him "no longer as a slave but more than a slave, as a beloved brother" (1:15). Surprisingly, as a modern commentator notes, "not a single word is devoted to the question whether the slave should be given freedom."[13] In other passages, Paul is more ambiguous about whether conversion to Christian faith requires emancipation: "Everyone should remain in the state in which he is called. Were you a slave when called? Never mind. But if you can gain your freedom, use it more" (1 Cor. 7:21–23). Although the thrust of the passage is to encourage acceptance of one's position, the possibility of gaining freedom is not ruled out; and in some cases it may even be a better use of one's faith than servitude.

The decisive issue is that, in the New Testament, social and political institutions are governed by conventions and prudence because the state and social order do not ultimately affect the dignity of a Christian (except for the family, whose monogamous and patriarchal character is required by the divinely created and natural order of things). Human dignity does not require external recognition because it rests on inner, spiritual freedom that depends, paradoxically, on becoming a new type of slave, "a slave of Christ" (1 Cor. 7:22). Unconditional submission to Christ as Lord and King—this demand alone is absolute; all other obligations (to one's nation, emperor, social class, the whole natural world, and even to one's family) are conditional. A new realm is opened up in everyone—the "innermost self" (Rom. 7:22); the "inner nature" (2 Cor. 4:16); the "hidden person of the heart" (1 Pet. 3:4)—which concerns the intimate question of the soul's relation to God. The inner realm is the real source of dignity in all persons because it means that something infinite is at stake in their life's choices: everyone has an immortal soul with an eternal destiny, which has at risk its eternal salvation or damnation.

Compared to the inner struggles of the soul against sin, the various forms of external obedience, while not matters of indifference, are of secondary importance. Thus, it is possible for biblical Christianity to uphold the dignity of man as a creature made in the image of God and redeemed by Christ while also admonishing obedience to created, natural, and conventional hierarchies.

Human Dignity in Patristic and Medieval Christianity

If we turn from the Bible to the Christian theology of the early Church and medieval period, we see continuities with the general hierarchical understanding of human dignity found in the Old and New Testaments. This should come as no surprise. The theologians of this period sought the help of reason to clarify and to explain the revealed truths of the Bible; and reason meant primarily classical Greek philosophy. Hence, the early Church Fathers turned to Plato and Neoplatonism, while the medieval Scholastics relied on Aristotle. In both cases, the classical Greek philosophers supported and even magnified the hierarchical teachings of the Bible. For the central thought of Plato and Aristotle is the idea of Nature as an intelligible order whose various parts can be ranked hierarchically according to their perfections as rational beings. When this idea was incorporated into the Christian faith, the main consequence was not to diminish hierarchies but to articulate them more precisely in terms of the essential attributes of the beings, forms, substances, or souls that make up the natural universe.

While this approach was difficult to apply to some phenomena, it seemed to provide a clear answer to the question of what constitutes man and his dignity: Man is an animal whose essential attribute is reason; hence, man's dignity derives from his existence as an intellectual substance or rational soul. The influence of this definition was such that St. Augustine could write in his commentaries on Genesis, as if it were self-evident, that "it is especially by reason of the mind that we understand that man was made to the image and likeness of God"; even "the erect form of the body" testifies to the fact that man is a "rational substance" because it enables him to look up and contemplate the heavens.[14] The crucial question is whether this philosophical-theological approach provides a new and improved understanding of human dignity.

Obviously, the momentous step of understanding the Bible in the light of Greek philosophy is fraught with dangers as well as possibilities. On the one hand, the Bible speaks of man in terms of the image, likeness, and form of God, which sounds like a Platonic approach. But the Bible seems to use such terms to avoid designating a set of qualities as the essential attributes of man, thereby precluding a Christian theory of human nature in the strict sense. Instead of focusing on essential attributes, the Bible presents man in terms of his relations to God: Originally man is closely related as the image of God; then he falls away; eventually the lost image of God may be restored through the redemptive sacrifice of Christ.[15] In this light, the Bible appears to be more interested in "soteriology" (the theory of salvation) than in "anthropology" (the theory of man).

On the other hand, the Bible does not forbid speculation about the essential attributes of man and even encourages it in the books of Wisdom and Ecclesiasticus. In addition, as I have argued, the biblical theory of salvation presupposes that the attribute of immortality is the lost image of God and that man in his present fallen state has a dual nature, both divine and sinful. Because of these complexities, we need to ask how the biblical view of human dignity was developed or changed by the incorporation of Greek philosophy into Christian theology. To simplify the answer, we shall limit ourselves to three points of comparison and a critical note raised by Eric Voegelin.

The first point concerns the claim of Plato and Aristotle that the natural universe is an intelligible or rational order. This implies that reason of some kind—*nous* or mind—pervades the entire universe and is not solely the preserve of man, although man is the only living animal with a rational soul capable of grasping (at least in part) the intelligibility of the world. One of the consequences of such a view is to lower the dignity of man by diminishing his uniqueness and permitting comparisons with other beings that might be more rational. Hence, Aristotle asserts (as quoted above) that "man is not the best thing in the universe . . . [although] it may be said that man is the best of the animals (*zoon*) . . . there are other things whose nature is more divine than man's: to take the most visible example, the things of which the celestial system is composed" (*Ethics*, 1141a21–1141b). For the Greek philosophers, in other words, reason pervades the entire universe in varying degrees of perfection, with man's reason somewhere near the middle—higher than other animals but lower than the heavenly bodies with their perfectly rational circular motion and lower still than the divine mind (God or the Good), which stands above but not outside of nature as the cause of intelligibility and motion in all things.

In turning to this scheme for help in understanding God's created order, Christian theologians could not accept the ranking of man below the heavenly bodies, because it contradicted the account of Genesis, which placed man at the peak of creation. As Christians, they held that man is the best thing in the natural universe. Yet, as a consequence of accepting the Greek philosophical view that the universe is a rational as well as a created order, many theologians accepted a slight diminution of man's unique status by acknowledging a variety of rational substances and rational principles in the universe as reflections of God's supreme rationality. As a result, they were willing to extend "the image and likeness of God" beyond man to other creatures and even to the entire natural universe.

The shift is explicitly marked in the Aristotelian Christianity of Thomas Aquinas, although it was deeply rooted in the Neoplatonic Christianity of the Church Fathers. In Aquinas, it follows from the technical distinction between things made in the "image" and those made in the "likeness" of God. An image, Aquinas says, is a copy of something, like a statue of a person, whereas a likeness is a vestige or trace of something, like the footprints of an animal (this distinction is apparently implied in the Hebrew words *tzelem* and *demuth*). Accordingly, "while in all creatures there is some kind of likeness to God, in the rational creature alone we find a likeness of *image* . . . whereas in other creatures we find a likeness by way of a *trace*" (*S. Th.*, I, 93.6; emphasis by Aquinas). Thus, rational creatures resemble God in knowing and understanding; while "other creatures do not understand, although we observe in them a certain trace of the Intellect that created them . . . For the fact that a creature has a modified and finite nature, proves that it proceeds from a principle, while its species points to the (mental) word of the maker" (ibid). In other words, rational creatures are closer to God because they are capable of understanding; but irrational creatures are nevertheless rational creations because God made them according to a plan or principle, giving them definite natures that are traces of his intellect.

Moreover, Aquinas claims that the whole hierarchical ordering of the universe is a likeness of God. In the *Summa Contra Gentiles,* he says it was God's "prerogative to induce His likeness into created things most perfectly . . . [but] there would not be a perfect likeness of God in the universe if all things were of one grade of being." Hence, God made "the diversity and inequality of created things" to actualize every possibility short of equality with himself and to show the goodness of creation in the ordering of diverse parts (II, 45.2–8). In similar fashion, St. Augustine speaks of the "goodness" of the created universe in all its parts, including, paradoxically, the existence of evil. Often, he says, we do not understand what the goodness of something might be; but we must trust, as a matter of faith, that creation is good. In a somewhat cryptic formulation, he says that nothing in the universe is inherently evil, only more or less good: "Evil is merely a name for the privation of good. There is a scale of value stretching from earthly to heavenly realities, from the visible to the invisible; and the inequality of these goods makes possible the existence of them all" (*City of God,* 11.23). What Augustine seems to mean is that the creation of the universe by God could not have occurred unless it were good, and a good creation requires an ordered hierarchy of unequal parts. Although human beings are special because of their rational natures and because we see "in ourselves an image of God, that is of the Supreme Trinity" (11.26), the whole universe, not only man, is a reflection of God in its goodness. Like the Bible, Aquinas and Augustine see man's dignity as comparative rather than absolute; but going beyond the Bible, they see God's likeness in the rational and hierarchical order of the entire universe.

The second major way that the ancient and medieval Christian theologians depart from the Bible follows from the first: Man is seen as a rational substance, but he is not the only nor even the highest one; in particular, the angels are rational substances of a higher order than man. Angels, of course, are found in both the Old and New Testaments as messengers of God. But they assume greater prominence in early and medieval Christian theology than in the Bible. They receive ontological status as rational beings without bodies or as minds separated from matter differentiated only by form, and they are given the important mission of divinizing the world and uplifting creation toward God.

The science of angels—"angelology" as some call it—may be hard
for people to take seriously today (although angels are making a come-
back in folk religion as well as in scientific searches for extraterrestrial
life, especially for forms of "higher" intelligence). Whatever one may
think of angelology as a metaphysical or empirical science, one must
acknowledge its significance for assessing the dignity of man: The existence of angels as higher forms of intelligence lowers the dignity of man
by one rank. As Aquinas bluntly asserts: "The dignity of angels sur-
passes that of men" (*S. Th.*, I, 59.3). The hierarchy of rational substances
thus proceeds from God to angels to man to irrational creatures.

This hierarchy is clearly an important part of patristic and medieval
theology. Indeed, St. Augustine feels compelled to include the creation
of angels in his account of the first day of creation; he sees them as forms
of invisible light that participate in the rational ordering of the visible
world, like the intelligible forms of Plato (*City of God*, 11.9). Aquinas
insists on the existence of angels for the perfection of the universe,
which requires intellectual or spiritual substances almost like God in
order to predominate over material substances and to draw the world
to God (*S. Th.*, I, 50.1–3). The effects of these spiritual beings on man
is both humbling and elevating: Man is diminished by comparison to
higher beings but also drawn upward by heavenly intermediaries of
God. According to the most influential work on angels, *The Celestial
Hierarchy* by the unknown pseudo-Dionysius of the early centuries A.D.,
this movement is the very purpose of hierarchies: "A hierarchy is a
sacred order . . . approximating as closely as possible to the divine . . .
for every member of the hierarchy, perfection consists in [being] uplifted to imitate God as far as possible" (3.1–3.2). In the Neoplatonic
Christianity of the author, the angels are necessary beings because God
is utterly transcendent and hidden, beyond all created being, yet the
unknown God also enters the known world, which requires the angels
as intermediary agents. Hence, God "first emerges from secrecy to revelation by way of mediation by these first powers" (13.4). The highest
order of angels (seraphim and cherubim) are the first to know God and
lovingly raise their inferiors; reciprocally, the "beings of lower ranks . . .
look upward to those intelligent beings of the first rank through
whom . . . they will be uplifted to the possible likeness of God"
(13.3–13.4). But the capacities for divinization vary, like the capacities

for absorbing and reflecting light, so each intellectual substance will be elevated "according to his measure" (*The Divine Names*, 4.2).

Whatever one may think about the existence of angelic beings (a possibility that cannot be dismissed as along as no one knows how mind relates to matter), one must at least acknowledge the power of believing in them: They have inspired some of the greatest works of "heavenly" beauty in Christian civilization, from the soaring luminosity of Gothic cathedrals to the celestial choir music of Palestrina and the *Panis Angelicus* to the lofty rhetoric of Lincoln's appeal to "the better angels of our nature." Without the hierarchical theory of rational substances, it is unlikely that these monuments to human dignity would exist.

The third major point about the dignity of man as a rational substance concerns politics: This notion is no more hospitable than the Bible to the principles of democracy and freedom. In fact, it may be less so, because it gives new sanctions to hierarchical structures in the social and political spheres. We should recall that the New Testament distinguishes between created, natural, and conventional hierarchies and indicates that most social and political institutions, except for the family and the church, fall into the category of conventional hierarchies. The realm of Caesar is distinguished from the realm of God, which means, on the simplest level, that the state or form of government and the arrangement of social classes are merely "human institutions"—their specific form is based on custom, agreement, and coercion—which nevertheless must be obeyed as instruments of God to restrain sinful men. In developing this teaching, Christian theologians strengthened such hierarchies by extending Paul's notion of a natural law written in the heart (Rom. 2:14–15) into the political realm.

For St. Augustine, the social and political hierarchies are part of the "tranquillity of order," which earthly cities strive to achieve in the fallen world. While never developing this notion into a full-blown theory of natural law, he describes it as a condition of "peace" where all things find their proper places according to "the law by which the natural order is governed" (*City of God*, 19.13). In Aquinas, a fully developed theory of natural law directs rational creatures toward virtue or the perfection of their natures and also provides sanctions for a hierarchical society. Accordingly, Aquinas says that the best form of government is a mixed regime combining elements of monarchy, aristocracy, and democracy—

"a kingdom wherein one is given the power to preside over all according to his virtue, while under him are others having governing powers according to their virtue, and yet a government of this kind is shared by all . . . because all are eligible to govern" (*S. Th.*, I-II, 105.1). While Augustine and Aquinas expect prudence to play a large role in politics, their natural norms provide more sanctions for political and social hierarchies than does the New Testament.

Moreover, even though their definition of man as a rational substance includes the notion of free will, their teachings do not prepare the way for modern liberal democracy based on individual rights. This point is important to understand because the language of the Scholastics on these matters can sometimes sound surprisingly like modern liberalism. For example, Aquinas states that man is "made to God's image, in so far as the image implies an intelligent being endowed with free-will and self-movement" (*S. Th.*, I-II, 1, Prologue). To some, this description may sound like the rational individual of Kantian liberalism who has dignity by virtue of his reason, freedom, and power of self-determination. Does it not follow that such an individual is a person, possessing rights, and that Thomism may evolve naturally into modern liberalism, making Thomas the first "Catholic Whig"? The answer that Thomas gives, both directly and indirectly, is that a rational being endowed with freedom and self-motion is not inherently a possessor of rights because reason does not have unconditional worth as an end-in-itself. Rather, reason has only conditional worth because it has an end beyond itself, namely, submission to a higher order of being and the attainment of man's last end, which is eternal happiness. Freedom, therefore, cannot be understood as a natural right to use reason according to formal procedures without specifying the end; freedom is only a conditional good that is lawful, right, or licit to the extent that it attains or at least seeks to attain reason's proper end.

Specifically, Thomas says, "Since man is said to be in the image of God by reason of his intellectual nature, he is most perfectly like God . . . in this, that God understands and loves Himself. Whereof we see that the image of God is in man in three ways. First, inasmuch as man possesses a natural aptitude for understanding and loving God . . . which consists in the very nature of the mind. Second, inasmuch as man actually or habitually knows and loves God, though imperfectly, and this image consists in the conformity of grace. Third, inasmuch as man knows and loves God perfectly, and this image consists in the likeness of glory . . . The first is found in all men, the second only in the just, the third only in the blessed" (*S. Th.*, I, 93.4). In other words, Aquinas sees the God-given capacities for reason, freedom, and self-motion as having an ultimate end beyond themselves, namely, intellectual apprehension of the good, which is God as well as the likeness of God in the whole created universe. Hence, there is no claim of autonomy for the rational will as there is in Kantian liberalism and no grounds for claiming that man is "born free," which is the premise of individual rights. Instead, man as a rational being made in the image of God implies the freedom to serve higher ends and leads to a hierarchy of human beings. The first level of the hierarchy recognizes our common humanity in the ordinary dignity of all rational creatures who possess in some fashion the desire to know the Creator; the second level includes those who attain some degree of that knowledge because they have received the faith through grace; the third includes only those who are blessed with glory because they will know and love God perfectly in the world-to-come.

These intellectual and spiritual distinctions, it must be emphasized, do not automatically translate into a political teaching for Aquinas—as if the saints should rule politically, as some Calvinists later argued. Aquinas recognizes the difference between the spiritual order and the temporal order, which means politics is determined in large measure by prudence applying natural law. Yet, the distinctions in the capacity for knowledge and love of God predispose Aquinas toward hierarchical rather than democratic models of authority in both the spiritual and temporal realms. In other words, the hierarchy of rational substances in the whole universe is paralleled by a hierarchy of human beings in the spiritual order as well as by a somewhat different hierarchy in the political order. Thus, human dignity is hierarchical; for God imparts his likeness and man receives God's likeness in varying degrees of perfection.

In assessing this view of human dignity, one could say many things, but perhaps the most pertinent is the cautionary note of Eric Voegelin. In *The Gospel and Culture*, he warns that "the history of Christianity is characterized by the separation of school theology from mystical and experiential theology."[16] Voegelin's concern is that the attempt by theologians to give doctrinal form to Christianity in terms of substances or essences inevitably leads to rigidity in the understanding of man and his relation to God. That is because humanity is not an essence but an experience, according to Voegelin; it is not the possession of attributes and faculties but openness to the mystical experience of transcendence in finite beings who are drawn toward the infinite divine ground of reality. This experience of living "in-between" the poles of existence is primary and universal, although it is expressed in different symbols by every civilization, indicating either healthy and balanced openness to transcendence or deformed and unbalanced closure.

In Voegelin's eyes, the two supreme expressions of openness are Platonic *eros,* which draws the human mind to the divine *nous,* and Christian-Pauline grace, in which God comes to man to sanctify humanity. Taken separately, the two are healthy. Indeed, the Christianity of the Gospels and Epistles, especially Paul's statement that in the Incarnation of Christ "the fullness of divine reality (*theotetes*) dwells bodily" (Col. 2:9), seems to Voegelin the most sublime expression of the divine presence in man.[17] Yet, when Greek philosophy and the Christian Incarnation are brought together in theological doctrines of the "hypostatic" union of two natures in one person and when man is defined as a type of intellectual substance, something bad happens: A distortion occurs in the original openness to the divine presence in Christ and among fellow men (*Gospel and Culture,* 153–58). The mystical experience of transcendence is cut off, replaced by hardened doctrines of "natures," "persons," and "substances" which reduce God and man to sets of attributes, eventually provoking the skeptical and destructive reactions of modern philosophy. In this assessment, Christian theology diminishes man's dignity and sows the seeds of modern secular ideologies.

Voegelin's advice, however, is not to jettison the theological enterprise but to use it properly, as did, he claims, the greatest Christian theologians of the patristic and medieval period. In his letter-essay, "On Christianity" (1953), he remarks that "the greatest value of Christian theology [is] as store of religious experiences amassed over a thousand years . . . analyzed and differentiated by Church Fathers and Scholastics in an extraordinary cooperative enterprise." In this period, theologians understood that "dogmatics is a symbolic web which explicates and differentiates religious experiences . . . not a rational system capable of being deduced from axioms . . . [hence] the insistence of Thomas that the Incarnation, Trinity, and other doctrines are rationally impene-

trable." Above all, Voegelin praises "the critical understanding of theological speculation . . . attained by Dionysius the Areopagite and by
Thomas Aquinas"; they recognized that "theology is the *analogia entis*"
[the analogy of being] . . . [in which] theological judgments are not
judgments in the sense of statements about the content of the world."[18]
While Voegelin undoubtedly errs in claiming that patristic and Scho-
lastic theology is a purely symbolic expression of experiences rather than
statements about reality (in the "analogy of being," verbal statements
refer to realities that point beyond themselves to more hidden realities),
he nevertheless raises the crucial point: The biblical understanding of
man as the image of God is distorted if the theological view of man as
a rational substance is taken too literally, and an anthropology or set of
qualities is substituted for man's mysterious relations with God.

As we shall see, however, the distortion of turning man into a
frozen being is less characteristic of ancient and medieval Christian theology than it is of modern theology. For the ancient hierarchical view
keeps ever-present in the conception of man the image of more perfect yet more mysterious realities, while modern theology tends to turn
man into a hardened substance—a "person" possessing absolute worth
and individual rights.

Human Dignity in Modern Christian Theology

To see at a glance the gulf separating the traditional hierarchical view
of human dignity from the modern democratic view, we need only survey a recent book, *Christianity and Democracy in Global Context* (1993).
With a foreword by Jimmy Carter and including articles from prominent spokespersons from many churches and nations, this book reveals
the broad consensus today among Protestants and Catholics about the
democratic implications of Christianity. The editor, John Witte, Jr.,
summarizes the general outlook with the observation that "Christianity
and democracy complement . . . [and] challenge each other" (12–13).
They complement each other because Christianity provides a spiritual
foundation for the democratic principles of equality and liberty, while
democracy offers a practical system of government that suits the Christian "concerns for human dignity and depravity." At the same time, the
two ideals challenge each other by restraining their worst tendencies.

Christianity checks the tendency of modern democracies to idolize progress, technology, materialism, inhuman industrialization, and the nihilistic consequences of purely secular freedom. Democracy checks the tendency of many Christian churches toward theocracy, hierarchicalism, and intolerant dogmatism. This overview offers a reassuring contemporary assessment of the relation between Christianity and democracy that the diverse figures of this volume—from former presidents to neoconservatives, feminists, Catholic and Anglican archbishops, as well as academic theologians—could embrace.[19]

Most of the contributors are aware, of course, that relations have not always been so smooth. Writing for the Protestant tradition, Witte admits that "the early Protestant reformers had little sympathy for democratic government. Martin Luther and Richard Hooker favored monarchy. Ulrich Zwingli and John Calvin favored aristocracy. Peter Ridman and Menno Simmons eschewed politics altogether" (5). Writing for the Catholic tradition, Brian Hehir and Roberto Papini acknowledge that the relation between Roman Catholicism and democracy was generally distrustful until the late nineteenth and twentieth centuries, when Popes Leo XIII and Pius XII began to accept qualified notions of natural rights.[20] Eventually John XXIII and the Second Vatican Council redefined religious liberty and embraced democratic human rights based on the "dignity of the human person" that subsequent popes have strongly endorsed (18–22, 50–54). The sweeping historical perspective presented by these authors is extremely illuminating because it shows how much the churches have changed in their attitudes toward democracy and human rights.

The principal reason for the change, we are told, is that, although earlier theologians and church leaders had little sympathy for democratic ideals, the Christian notions of "person and society . . . were filled with democratic implications" that gradually and painfully came to be recognized. The crucial concept is the *human person,* which the authors of this volume (and many beyond it) embrace as the link between traditional Christianity and the modern ideals of democracy and human rights. As Wolfgang Huber argues, democracy and human rights are based on "an image of human persons who are gifted with an inalienable dignity and who live their lives in responsible freedom"; this notion, he claims, is "clearly linked to basic assumptions of Christian anthropology . . . [and is] indebted to Christian sources" (35). In other words, the original faith of Christianity contained a notion of the equal dignity of persons that was only dimly grasped, and sometimes even suppressed, by its early leaders; through progressive evolution, however, the democratic essence of the person was recognized, enabling the Christian tradition to nurture and inspire such modern political ideals as inalienable rights, liberty of conscience, and constitutional checks on state power (35). This development makes it possible to see a kind of inner affinity between the Christian view of the person and the modern democratic personality. In the words of Jacques Maritain, the democratic ideal has become "the profane name of the Christian ideal" (55).

While the authors do not explain in detail how the democratic view of human dignity triumphed among Christians (they simply record its progress and take its victory for granted), many factors might be cited: the influence of the Protestant Reformation and its notions of individual conscience and covenanting communities; the influence of neo-Thomistic ideas of popular sovereignty developed by Jesuits and Dominicans; the impact of the Enlightenment and its critical attitude toward all authorities as well as the rationalistic religions it spawned; the impact of the democratic revolutions in America, France, and Russia on church politics; the arguments against colonialism and slavery developed by Las Casas and the Quakers; the tactical shifts by Catholics in the nineteenth century on the issues of religious liberty and workers' rights, eventually codified in the Second Vatican Council; the Christian reactions to totalitarianism in the twentieth century. All of these movements chipped away at the deeply rooted hierarchical patterns of thought stemming from the Bible and from traditional theology and contributed to the opening of Christianity to democratic vistas. Yet, in the last analysis, I would argue that the decisive factor has been the intellectual movements growing out of the Enlightenment, especially the philosophy of freedom developed by Immanuel Kant and various philosophical currents growing out of Kant, including Hegelianism, phenomenology, existentialism, and neo-Kantianism.

I single out the Kantian philosophy of freedom as the decisive factor because it seems to match most closely the contemporary Christian concern for the rights and dignity of the person and to account most precisely for the terminology of personhood and personality that Christians now employ. The change can be seen in the new understanding of the image of God, which no longer reflects the traditional hierarchy of being and perfection with its sometimes harsh implications of judging according to created, natural, conventional, and ecclesiastical hierarchies. Instead, the image of God now means the infinite worth of every human being as a "person"—as a moral agent claiming respect as a matter of right and capable of determining his or her own identity. Consequently, the *Imago Dei* now includes a moral imperative to establish democratic political structures where the rights of persons are fully recognized and where all share equally in the goods of the world and indeed in the blessings of the afterlife (not excluding the democratic hope that everyone will be saved). If this account is accurate, then contemporary Christianity is essentially *Kantian Christianity*. For Kant is the one who took the decisive step in defending the absolute worth or dignity of all rational beings, calling them "persons" as opposed to "objects" or "things" and demanding that they be treated as ends rather than as mere means and endowing them with inalienable human rights. Whether Kant applied the dignity and rights of persons to man alone or to other rational beings in the universe is somewhat unclear, but his notion has subsequently been developed into a powerful philosophy of human freedom by many scholars and theologians who have profoundly influenced the Christian concept of human dignity.

One reason why Kant's philosophy of freedom has appealed to Christian theologians is that it provides a modern way of defending human dignity while maintaining important points of continuity with the tradition. In the Bible, the dignity of man as a creature made in the image of God refers primarily to lost immortality and to the possibility of regaining immortality through Christ. Kant's idea of dignity preserves a connection with immortality by stipulating it as a postulate of practical reason—as a logical assumption of morality. But Kant's most important continuity with tradition lies in the claim that human dignity applies to rational beings, though Kant radically redefines the essence of rationality. Traditionally it meant a natural inclination toward intellectual apprehension of the Good, which made theoretical wisdom or contemplative knowledge of God and God's creation the highest end of reason. For Kant, theoretical knowledge is impossible because of reason's inherent limitations, which leaves only the practical goal of knowing and realizing morality. By incorporating Kant into Christianity, modern theologians find continuity with biblical, Augustinian, and Thomistic themes about eternal life and the greatest good, while developing a new understanding of Christian ethics that raises moral and practical concerns to the highest priority, especially the imperatives of social justice and perpetual peace based on respect for the dignity of persons and their human rights.

If this observation is correct, then most contemporary versions of Christianity are best understood as combinations of Thomism and Kantianism (the Catholic model) or of Augustinianism and Kantianism (the Protestant model). The key to such combinations, I believe, is the changing notion of the "person." In patristic and medieval Christian theology, person was a *metaphysical* term meaning an "individual substance of a rational nature," which was applied almost exclusively to the three Persons of the Trinity. In recent years, person has been developed into a *moral* term applied to human beings, meaning rational and free agents who possess inherent dignity and inalienable rights along the lines described by Kant. While some theologians (especially Catholic neo-Thomists) see a fairly smooth transition from the metaphysical to the moral dimensions of the person—arguing that "person" describes not merely a type of "substance" but also a type of "relation" between beings, including self-giving love—I think that the equation of moral relations with respecting the *rights of persons* moves outside of the sphere of Thomism and even of Christian charity into the realm of Kantian liberalism.[21] To illustrate the point, let me cite some examples of this subtle but highly significant development in modern Christian theology.

In Catholicism, one can see it in the towering figure of Jacques Maritain. He is the most influential spokesman for Catholic "personalism"—the dominant brand of Catholic theology in the twentieth century among scholars and church leaders (espoused in one fashion or another not only by Maritain but also by Emmanuel Mounier, Gabriel Marcel, Heinrich Rommen, John Courtney Murray, and Michael Novak as well as by Popes John XXIII, Paul VI, and John Paul II). Maritain took the concept of the "person" from Thomistic metaphysics and turned it into a theory of the human personality that combined the transcendent longings and social nature of traditional Thomism with the autonomous agency of a free person who possesses a host of economic, social, and political rights. Those rights, which Maritain helped to inscribe in the United Nations' Universal Declaration of Human Rights, are virtually identical to those of Kantian liberalism—freedom of conscience, the right to participate in the decisions of society, property rights, as well as rights to social security and decent standards of living. Maritain's synthesis of traditional Thomistic natural law and modern human rights culminated in his theory of "personalist democracy" as the alternative to secular individualism and Marxist collectivism.

In similar fashion, John Courtney Murray combined Thomistic natural law and modern natural rights to develop a new defense of religious freedom based on the "dignity of the human person." These currents deeply influenced the thinking of Pope John XXIII and the Second Vatican Council. In his encyclical *Pacem in Terris* (1963), which set the tone for the Council, John XXIII declared, "Every human being is a person; his nature is endowed with intelligence and free will. By virtue of this he has rights and duties of his own, flowing directly from his very nature, which are therefore universal, inviolable, and inalienable" (par. 9). While the language of Thomas is still present in the encyclical, the unmistakable Kantian elements are also there and sometimes predominate, as in the statements that "by the natural law every human being has the right to respect for his person" (12) and "from the dignity of the human person there also arises the right to carry on economic activities" (20). The language and sentiments of Pope John are also evident in the documents of the Council, such as the Declaration on Religious Freedom and the Constitution on the Church in the Modern World, which attempt to adapt church teachings to the growing "sense of the dignity of the human person [that] has been impressing itself . . . on the consciousness of contemporary man" (DRF, 1). In the years since Vatican II, the dignity and rights of the human person have been restated many times by Pope John Paul II, beginning with *The Acting Person* (1977) and continuing in several encyclicals and even in his popular writings, such as *Crossing the Threshold of Hope*, where the pope says his whole interest in "man as person" and the "dignity of the person" or "the personalistic principle" arose as "an attempt to translate the commandment of love into the language of philosophical ethics . . . of Kantian ethics" (200–201). Yet, as often as the pope speaks like Kant, he also appeals to Thomas Aquinas. Hence, in *The Splendor of Truth*, he argues that freedom must serve the end of truth and that conscience must submit to the objective order of the natural moral law (60), where natural law commands the love of God and respect for the dignity of the human person. The goal of Pope John Paul II, it seems to me, is to

develop a synthesis of Thomism and a Kantian version of phenomenology that tips the scales in favor of traditional natural law duties over
modern natural rights.

In Protestant theology, the lines of development are not as clear
as in Catholicism due to sectarian divergences. Moreover, Augustine
is usually the preferred Doctor of Theology among Protestants rather
than Thomas, which means that theological innovations tend to grow
out of the doctrine of grace rather than out of natural law, producing
more amorphous notions of "personhood" than Catholic "personalism."
Nevertheless, one can find cases that closely parallel developments in
Catholicism. For example, Martin Luther King, Jr.'s powerful "Letter
from a Birmingham Jail" (1963) develops the "higher law" of Augustine
and Aquinas by adding a Kantian and existential notion of human dignity. As King says, "An unjust law is a code that is out of harmony with
the moral law. To put it in the terms of St. Thomas Aquinas: An unjust
law is a human law that is not rooted in eternal law and natural law. Any
law that *uplifts human personality* is just. Any law that *degrades human
personality* is unjust. All segregation statutes are unjust because segregation distorts the soul and *damages the personality*. It gives the seg-
regator a false sense of superiority and the segregated a false sense
of inferiority. Segregation, to use the terminology of the Jewish philosopher Martin Buber, substitutes an 'I-it' relationship for an 'I-thou'
relationship and ends up relegating *persons to the status of things*"
(121, emphasis added). It is impossible not to hear in Martin Luther
King's formulation another version of Christian personalism, combining
Thomistic higher law with Kant's notion of treating people as persons
rather than as things (mediated by Martin Buber's Jewish existential
personalism, which distinguishes "thou" from "it" exactly the way that
Kant distinguishes "persons" from "things").[22]

In another variation of modern Christianity, Glenn Tinder develops a Lutheran strand of Augustinianism by combining it with elements of Kantian and existential freedom. In *The Political Meaning of
Christianity,* Tinder argues that the central message of Christianity is
respect for the "exalted individual"—respect for the infinite worth and
dignity of all individuals because of their unique and irreplaceable identities. Everyone is exalted, he says, because God commands "you to do
what your authentic being or destiny requires. God commands you to
be truly yourself" (208). This concept, Tinder argues, is the spiritual

center of Western politics and the only sound moral basis of liberal democratic rights because it contains the moral imperative that "governments be considerate, egalitarian, and universalist" (13, 178, 203). In other words, the love and respect for the authentic destiny that God has called each one of us to be leads to the political conclusion that "Christianity implies democracy" as the only form of government worthy of human dignity (178).[23]

What is fascinating about these trends in Christian theology is the high degree of common ground that Protestants and Catholics have found in certain features of Kantian liberalism and how both have converged with tendencies in secular liberal philosophy. For secular liberalism today is also powerfully influenced by Kantian and neo-Kantian ideas of "equal concern and respect" for every human being.[24] The crucial difference, of course, is that most secular theories today deny that there is any foundation for human dignity except for radical autonomy, while Kantian Christians always bring human dignity back to a foundation in the *Imago Dei*. But the *Imago Dei* has now been given a new twist, which includes the ethical imperative to affirm the rights and dignity of the self-defining person.

Conclusion: Which View of Human Dignity Is Best?

Having surveyed three views of human dignity, I would like to conclude by attempting to make some comparative judgments. For several important reasons, I think that the modern version of human dignity—the Kantian-Christian view—is the least satisfactory of the three and needs to be reconsidered in the light of the biblical and the medieval views, even if this conflicts with some of the most cherished convictions of the contemporary world.

The main problem with the modern view can be stated quite simply: It overstates the dignity of man, both collectively as a species and individually as persons. Lurking behind much of modern Christianity is the fear that modern science has given us a cosmos that consists of dumb matter, silently and indifferently obeying the mathematical laws of physics without any sign of God's Providence or Nature's benevolence. In such a universe, man alone has dignity—a dignity that is absolute or infinitely precious (as in the principle that human life, as mere biological existence, is sacred). Yet even Pascal, who often resembles Kant in speaking of the dignity of man in the indifferent universe of modern science, reminds us that "there are perfections in nature to show that she is the image of God and imperfections to show that she is no more than His image" (*Pensees,* #934). Following Pascal's thought (which in this passage is more medieval than modern), I would argue that it makes more sense to conceive of man not as an absolutely unique being in the cosmos but as the highest creature on a hierarchy of perfection in which all of nature participates—a universe in which all beings partake to some degree in the likeness and goodness of God (and that may also include mysterious beings that equal or surpass humans as intelligent beings).

Some modern environmentalists have begun to push Christianity in this direction, diminishing the absolute uniqueness of man by conceiving of the human species as part of an interconnected and self-adjusting natural order, thereby balancing one-sided Kantianism in which man alone possesses dignity and one-sided scientism in which nature is purely raw material for mastery. But environmentalists often err in losing sight of human distinctiveness, not to mention human superiority, in an indiscriminate pantheism where everything is equally sacred. A more balanced view is that nature is a created order of God, the whole of which is a likeness of God in its vastness, age, complexity, and intelligible order but which also points to man as its peak, the rational creature made in the image of God. Yet, the justification for that ranking remains mysterious, since no one can prove conclusively that mind or intelligence had to appear for the completion of the universe. Man's intelligence appears to us as a kind of perfection, but we have no idea if this is really why God favors man with his revelation and the possibility of eternal life. Hence, human dignity depends in the last analysis on our mysterious election by God and only secondarily on our rational souls; in such a world, human dignity is a type of comparative ranking in a divinely created hierarchy of beings rather than the absolute worth of an absolutely unique being.

A second problem with the modern Kantianized version of Christianity is that it tends to equate the dignity of man with the rights of an autonomous being rather than with a soul that is both divine and sinful and that needs to be elevated by subordinating the personality to a higher order of being and even to human hierarchies. This traditional idea is wholly compatible with Christianity, despite its disfavor in the modern world. For, contrary to the belief of many modern Christians and even some anti-Christians (like Nietzsche), Christianity is not a purely democratic or egalitarian religion; it is a hierarchical religion. Of course, Christianity often opposes the hierarchies of the world (as measured by birth, wealth, power, talent, and physical beauty) and therefore often conflicts with the world, as it did in pagan Rome. But Christianity opposes worldly hierarchies with hierarchies of its own; and it does not have as its primary mission the abolition of worldly hierarchies but merely their recognition as the inescapable follies of a fallen world where "man judges by appearances while God judges the heart." As the lives of the saints and the practices of the most devout religious and monastic orders have shown, the soul cannot be elevated without suppressing the personality or the autonomous will of the person through the discipline of prayer, work, silence, service, song, suffering, and obedience to hierarchies.

Precisely because it is hierarchical, however, Christianity is not the absolute enemy of democracy in the secular or temporal realm—that is, in the realm of politics (which also includes economics and social class). For according to the proper understanding of the hierarchy of ends, the temporal realm is of secondary importance compared to the spiritual realm and is therefore largely governed by prudence or prudential considerations. Yet, the secondary status of politics does not mean that it is a matter of indifference. It means that politics is generally distinguished from spiritual matters and should focus on the mundane but necessary and difficult business of maintaining stable order and national security, punishing the wicked, inculcating decent moral habits to sustain responsible freedom and justice, cultivating a certain kind of civic piety, and, above all, "doing no harm" (that is, not forcing citizens to be immoral or impious).

Kantian Christianity confuses this point by turning spiritual duties into political rights—by making charity for our neighbors a matter of respecting their rights and empowering people to claim their rights. But charity is of a different order than justice, however justice is conceived, because charity is sacrificial love and therefore is not owed or deserved like justice. Moreover, charity is required by divine law; but no particular political regime—neither monarchy nor democracy nor even theocracy—is required by divine law in Christianity. Up until the seventeenth century (and even up to the twentieth century), most Christian theologians understood this to mean that a variety of different regimes could be legitimate, depending on the circumstances, as long as the relatively modest goals of the earthly city could be achieved. Hierarchical regimes—monarchy or mixed regimes—were thought to be most suitable on prudential grounds for promoting order, moral virtue, and a certain degree of civic piety.

Following this traditional approach, a case could be made today on prudential grounds for all constitutionally limited regimes, including constitutional democracy or republicanism. The crucial question in the contemporary world, however, should not be confined to the issue of establishing stable order and responsible freedom but must emphatically raise the issue of "doing no harm." For today's democracies are closely tied to ideologies of rights and empowerment that often coerce citizens, either through the state or through social pressure that imposes a degraded culture, to be immoral and impious. If that is so, then democratic regimes would not pass the prudential test, and hierarchical regimes might be more justified. Serious proponents of Kantianized Christianity are certainly aware of the danger of exalting rights about religious duties, but they often seem inconsistent because they promote and at the same time condemn the culture of rights. The challenge of our age is therefore to combine a hierarchical view of human dignity in the realm of Christian spirituality (which includes the church and the family) with a qualified view of the democratic political order that is guided by sober prudence rather than by Kantian rights. If we can achieve that delicate balance, we will have made an important contribution to defending the true and authentic dignity of man.

Notes

1. Reinhold Niebuhr, *The Nature and Destiny of Man,* vol. 1, *Human Nature* (New York: Scribner's Sons, 1941, 1964), ch. 6, "Man as Image of God and as Creature," pp. 150–78; also 14–15, 55.

2. Quoted from Voegelin's "The Drama of Humanity" and "Siger de Brabant" in Ellis Sandoz, "Medieval Rationalism or Mystic Philosophy? Reflections on the Strauss-Voegelin Correspondence," in *Faith and Political Philosophy: The Correspondence between Leo Strauss and Eric Voegelin, 1934–1964,* trans. and ed. Peter

Emberley and Barry Cooper (University Park, Pa.: Pennsylvania State University Press, 1993), 309, 318.

3. John Paul II, *Centesimus Annus: The Social Teaching of the Church, Encyclical Letter of His Holiness on the One Hundreth Anniversary of Rerum Novarum,* Vatican trans. (Sherbrooke, Quebec: Editions Paulines, 1991), par. 11; also 22, 44.

4. *The Rights of Man,* in *The Thomas Paine Reader,* ed. Michael Foot and Isaac Kramnick (Harmondsworth, Eng.: Penguin Books, 1987), 216.

5. For a strong statement of the American faith, see Ellis Sandoz, "Philosophical and Religious Dimensions of the American Founding," *The Intercollegiate Review* 30:2 (Spring 1995): 27–42. See especially 36–39 for a summary of the Founders' view: "Liberty is . . . a natural trait which reflects the supernatural One whose image man is . . . Liberty is thus God-given . . . To live [under tyranny] is to abandon both God and our true selves . . . and [to] mutilate the divine image that animates the noble conception of man and reality reflected in Psalm 8, which is rightly called the Magna Carta of humanity . . . It is from such a perspective, one emphatically open to the horizon of being, that the ringing lines of the Declaration of Independence are to be . . . understood . . . [as well as] the Constitution and Bill of Rights."

6. Umberto Cassuto, *A Commentary on the Book of Genesis,* part 2, trans. Israel Abrahams (Jerusalem: Magnes Press, 1984), 127. See also Pope John Paul II, *The Gospel of Life,* par. 39, which examines this passage in Genesis.

7. For a fuller elaboration of the biblical view of environmentalism, see Ernest Fortin, "The Bible Made Me Do It: Christianity, Science, and the Environment," *The Review of Politics* 57:2 (Spring 1995): 197–224.

8. See Thomas L. Pangle, "The Hebrew Bible's Challenge to Political Philosophy: Some Introductory Reflections," in *Political Philosophy and the Human Soul: Essays in Memory of Allan Bloom,* ed. Michael Palmer and Thomas L. Pangle (Lanham, Md.: Rowman and Littlefield, 1995), 76–77.

9. Hence, Paul continues with the thought: "Does not nature itself teach you that for a man to wear long hair is degrading to him, but if a woman has long hair, it is her pride?" (1 Cor. 11:14).

10. The hierarchical character of the church is ordained before Paul in the words of Christ that establish the Apostles as authorities, not only explicitly in Matthew 16 where Christ selects Peter as head of the church but also more subtly in Luke and Matthew, where Christ indicates privileged knowledge for the disciples: "To you it has been given to know the secrets of the kingdom of God; but for others, they are in parables so that . . . they may not understand" (Luke 8:9–10; Matt. 13:11).

11. The only exceptions in the New Testament to accepting conventional class relations are James 2:1–8, which condemns showing "partiality" for the rich over the poor and even challenges some of the status symbols of the rich, although the

main point is to assert that the poor of the world are closer to God and "heirs of the kingdom"; also Acts 4:32–5:11, which describes an experiment in communal sharing of property among early Christians; the wider application of this experiment, however, is unclear because it involved separation by a small number from Roman society under the strict authoritarian direction of Peter and the Apostles; it also seems to have failed due to hoarding, never to be tried again.

12. Orlando Patterson, *Freedom in the Making of Western Civilization* (New York: Basic Books, 1991), vol. 1, ch. 17–19, pp. 304–44.

13. Eduard Lohse, *A Commentary on the Epistles to the Colossians and to Philemon,* trans. William R. Poehlmann and Robert J. Karris (Philadelphia: Fortress Press, 1971), 206.

14. St. Augustine, "Two Books on Genesis against the Manichees" and "On the Literal Interpretation of Genesis: An Unfinished Book," in *St. Augustine on Genesis, The Fathers of the Church,* vol. 84, trans. Roland J. Teske, S.J. (Washington, D.C.: Catholic University of America Press, 1991), 76, 186. Augustine was undoubtedly influenced by Ambrose, who notes in his commentary on Genesis that man's creation in the image of God consists in the possession of a spiritual "soul" as well as a body in erect posture for looking upward. Saint Ambrose, *Hexameron (Creation), Paradise, and Cain and Abel, The Fathers of the Church,* vol. 42, trans. John J. Savage (New York: Fathers of the Church, 1961), 253–83.

15. For an account of the two basic ways of explaining the Image of God— the "substantialist" (in terms of attributes, qualities, and faculties) and the "relational" (in terms of relations with God and the world), see Douglas J. Hall, *Imaging God: Dominion as Stewardship* (Grand Rapids, Mich.: Eerdmans, 1986), 88–108. For the difficulty of finding a theory of rights among the attributes or relations, see Kieran Cronin, *Rights and Christian Ethics* (Cambridge: Cambridge University Press, 1992), 253–66.

16. Eric Voegelin, "The Gospel and Culture," in *Faith and Political Philosophy: The Correspondence between Leo Strauss and Eric Voegelin, 1934–1964* (University Park, Pa.: Pennsylvania State University Press, 1993), 164.

17. Whether this is an adequate understanding of Christ and the Incarnation is a matter of considerable controversy among Voegelin scholars. See Eugene Webb, "Eric Voegelin's Theory of Revelation," and Thomas J. J. Altizer, "A New History and a New but Ancient God? Voegelin's *The Ecumenic Age,*" in *Eric Voegelin's Thought: A Critical Appraisal,* ed. Ellis Sandoz (Durham: Duke University Press, 1982), 157–88.

18. Eric Voegelin, "On Christianity," letter to Alfred Schutz (1 January 1953), in *The Philosophy of Order: Essays on History, Consciousness, and Politics,* ed. Peter J. Optiz and Gregor Sebba (Stuttgart: Lett-Cotta, 1981), 449–57.

19. The impressive list of contributors to *Christianity and Democracy in a Global Context,* ed. John Witte, Jr. (Boulder, Colo.: Westview Press, 1993) includes

such distinguished figures as former President Jimmy Carter, Archbishop Desmond M. Tutu, Catholic Archbishop of Panama Marcos McGrath, Father Richard John Neuhaus, as well as scholars such as Bryan Hehir, Jean Bethke Elshtain, Paul E. Sigmund, and Harold J. Berman.

20. For a fascinating account of the seemingly unthinking way that individual rights were incorporated into Leo's famous encyclical, see Ernest Fortin, "'Sacred and Inviolable': *Rerum Novarum* and Natural Rights," *Theological Studies* 53:2 (June 1992): 203–33.

21. See W. Norris Clarke, S.J., *Explorations in Metaphysics: Being, God, Person* (Notre Dame: University of Notre Dame Press, 1994), ch. 10, "Person, Being, and St. Thomas." Clarke emphasizes the need to develop the Thomistic person from a static substance to a dynamic relation among beings that includes self-communication to others and self-giving love; but Clarke seems oblivious to the whole dimension of political rights that Catholic theology has imputed to the person, which is not in Thomas and must be imported from Kant.

22. Martin Luther King, Jr., "Letter from a Birmingham Jail," in *What Country Have I? Political Writings by Black Americans,* ed. Herbert J. Storing (New York: St. Martin's Press, 1970), 117–31.

23. Glenn Tinder, *The Political Meaning of Christianity: An Interpretation* (Baton Rouge: Louisiana State University Press, 1989).

24. For this convergence, see the volume *Catholicism and Liberalism: Contributions to American Public Philosophy,* ed. R. Bruce Douglass and David Hollenbach (Cambridge: Cambridge University Press, 1994); Paul E. Sigmund notes the convergence on p. 235.

CHAPTER FOUR

Between Sanctity and Depravity: Human Dignity in Protestant Perspective

JOHN WITTE, JR.

Human Dignity as "Ur-Principle"

"A sense of the dignity of the human person has been impressing itself more and more deeply on the consciousness of contemporary man," Pope Paul VI declared in his preface to *Dignitatis Humanae* (1965). "And the demand is increasingly made that men should act on their own judgment, enjoying and making use of a responsible freedom, not driven by coercion but motivated by a sense of duty."[1]

This was a historic statement about human dignity, signaling a momentous swing in the pendulum of world opinion. Only two decades before, the world had stared in horror into Hitler's death camps and Stalin's gulags, where all sense of humanity and dignity had been brutally sacrificed. In response, the world had seized anew on the ancient concept of human dignity, claiming this as the "ur-principle" of a new world order.[2] The Universal Declaration of Human Rights of 1948 opened its preamble with what would become classic words: "recognition of the inherent dignity and of the equal and inalienable rights of all members of the human family is the foundation of freedom, justice, and peace in the world."[3]

By the mid-1960s, church and state alike had translated this general principle of human dignity into concrete human rights precepts. In *Dignitatis Humanae* and several other documents produced during and after the Second Vatican Council (1962–1965), the Roman Catholic Church took some of the first decisive steps. Every person, the church now taught, is created by God with "dignity, intelligence and free will . . . and has rights flowing directly and simultaneously from his very nature."[4] Such rights include the right to life and adequate standards of living, to moral and cultural values, to religious activities, to assembly and association, to marriage and family life, and to various social, political, and economic benefits and opportunities. The church emphasized the religious rights of conscience, worship, assembly, and education, calling them the "first rights" of any civic order. The church also stressed the need to balance individual and associational rights, particularly those involving the church, family, and school. Governments everywhere were encouraged to create conditions conducive to the realization and protection of these inviolable rights and encouraged to root out discrimination, whether social or cultural, whether based on sex, race, color, social distinction, language, or religion.[5] Within a decade, various ecumenical groups, some Protestants, and even a few Orthodox Christian groups crafted comparable comprehensive declarations on human rights—albeit with varying emphases on the concept of human dignity.[6]

Not only the world's churches but also the United Nations and several nation-states issued a number of landmark documents on human dignity and human rights in the 1960s. Foremost among these were the two great international covenants promulgated by the United Nations in 1966. Both these covenants took as their starting point the "inherent dignity" and "the equal and inalienable rights of all members of the human family" and the belief that all such "rights derive from the inherent dignity of the human person."[7] The International Covenant on Economic, Social, and Cultural Rights (1966) posed as essential to human dignity the rights to self-determination, subsistence, work, welfare, security, education, and various other forms of participation in cultural life. The International Covenant on Civil and Political Rights (1966) set out a long catalog of rights to life and to security of person and property, freedom from slavery and cruelty, basic civil and criminal procedural protections, rights to travel and pilgrimage, freedoms of religion, expression, and assembly, rights to marriage and family life, and freedom from discrimination on grounds of race, color, sex, language, and national origin. Other international and domestic instruments issued in the later 1960s took particular aim at racial, religious, and gender discrimination in education, employment, social welfare programs, and other forms and forums of public life—viewing such discrimination as a fundamental betrayal of the "dignity and equality inherent in all human beings."[8]

So matters stood up to 1970. Today, the concept of human dignity has become ubiquitous to the point of cliché—a moral trump frayed by heavy use, a general principle harried by constant invocation. From 1970 to 2000, there were more than 1,200 books and 11,000 scholarly articles on dignity published in English alone. We now read regularly of the dignity of animals, plants, and nature; the dignity of luxury, pleasure, and leisure; the dignity of poverty, pain, and imprisonment; the dignity of identity, belonging, and difference; the dignity of ethnic, cultural, and linguistic purity; the dignity of sex, gender, and sexual preference; the dignity of aging, dying, and death. At the same time, the corpus of human rights has become swollen to the point of eruption—with many recent rights claims no longer anchored in universal norms of human dignity but aired as special aspirations of an individual or a group. We now hear regularly of the right to peace, health, and beauty; the right to rest, holidays, and work breaks; the right to work, development, and economic expansion; the right to abortion, suicide, and death; and a whole host of special rights claims of women, children, workers, immigrants, refugees, prisoners, minorities, indigenous peoples, and many others.[9]

On the one hand, the current ubiquity of the principle of human dignity testifies to its universality. And the constant proliferation of human rights precepts speaks to their power to inspire new hope for many desperate persons and peoples around the world. Moreover, the increased pervasiveness of these norms is partly a function of emerging globalization. Since the first international documents on human dignity and human rights were issued, many new voices and values have joined the global dialogue—especially those from Africa, Asia, and Latin America, and from various Buddhist, Confucian, Hindu, Islamic, and Traditional communities. It is simple ignorance to assume that the first international documents were truly universal statements on human dignity and human rights. The views of Christians, Jews, and Enlightenment exponents dominated them.[10] And it is simple arrogance to assume that the 1940s through the 1960s were the golden age of human dignity and human rights. Such theological and legal constructions are in need of constant reformation. The recent challenges of the South and the East to the prevailing Western paradigm of human dignity and human rights might well be salutary.

On the other hand, the very ubiquity of the principle of human dignity today threatens its claims to universality. And the very proliferation of new human rights threatens their long-term effectiveness for doing good. Human dignity needs to be assigned some limits if it is to remain a sturdy foundation for the edifice of human rights. Human rights need to be founded firmly on human dignity and other moral principles lest they devolve into a gaggle of wishes and wants. Fairness commands as broad a definition of human dignity as possible, so that no legitimate human good is excluded and no legitimate human rights claim is foreclosed. But prudence counsels a narrower definition of human dignity, so that not every good becomes part of human dignity, and not every aspiration becomes subject to human rights vindication.

The task of defining the appropriate ambit of human dignity and human rights today must be a multidisciplinary, multireligious, and multicultural exercise. Many disciplines, religions, and cultures around the globe have unique sources and resources, texts and traditions that speak to human dignity and human rights. Some endorse dignity and rights with alacrity and urge their expansion into new arenas. Others demur, and urge their reform and restriction. It is essential that each community be allowed to speak with its own unique accent, to work with its own distinct methods on human dignity and human rights—that the exercise be multi- rather than interdisciplinary, interreligious, and intercultural in character. It is also essential, however, that each of these disciplines, religions, and cultures develops a capacity for bilingualism—an ability to speak with insiders and outsiders alike about their unique understanding of the origin, nature, and purpose of human dignity and human rights.

This volume of essays by scholars from various confessions and professions is precisely the kind of exercise that is currently needed. Happily, it is of a piece with a number of other important new studies that have appeared at this turn of the millennium by Jewish, Muslim, Confucian, Buddhist, and Hindu scholars working on issues of human dignity and human rights with their own texts and on their own terms.[11]

My assignment is to test the meaning and take the measure of human dignity in the Protestant tradition. My argument is that the Protestant tradition has a deep and distinctive understanding of human dignity, which has had and can still have a monumental influence on the understanding of human rights. In my view, the essence of human dignity lies in the juxtaposition of human depravity and human sanctity. Human dignity is something of a divine fulcrum that keeps our depravity and sanctity in balance. The essence of human freedom is our right and duty to serve God, neighbor, and self, and to do so with the ominous assurance of divine judgment. Human freedom is the divine calling that keeps our individuality and community in balance.

This understanding of human dignity and freedom, I argue, was already adumbrated in Martin Luther's famous little tract, *Freedom of a Christian* (1520). Luther's tract was something of a Protestant *Dignitatis Humanae* in its day, an enduring theological statement on the essence of human dignity and human freedom. Several theological teachings in this little tract were filled with radical political implications. While Luther did not draw out these implications, a number of later Protestants did, eventually rendering Protestantism a formidable force for the construction of modern Western human rights theories and laws. The last part of this essay reflects on the enduring efficacy of Luther's cardinal insights for our understanding of human dignity and human rights.

It must be stressed that I am presenting only one Protestant stream of reflection on human dignity, albeit a deep and enduring one. Other Protestants over the centuries have taken their departure more directly from those biblical texts that Robert Kraynak's essay herein so ably highlights—that persons were created in the "image of God," that they were made "a little lower than the angels," that they may partake of the universal spiritual dignity of Christ. Such Protestant views of human dignity tend to resonate more closely with prevailing Patristic, Catholic, and Humanist constructions, and today are considerably better known and more frequently proffered, especially in ecumenical discussions.[12] My rendering of the Protestant teaching on human dignity is not meant to deprecate these other Protestant contributions but to complement them.

Saint and Sinner, Priest and King

Martin Luther's *Freedom of a Christian* (1520) was one of the defining documents of the Protestant Reformation, and it remains one of the classic tracts of the Protestant tradition still today.[13] Written on the eve of his excommunication from the church, this was Luther's last ecumenical gesture toward Rome before making his incendiary exit. Much of the tract was written with a quiet gentility and piety that belied the heated polemics of the day and Luther's own ample perils of body and soul. Luther dedicated the tract to Pope Leo X, adorning it with a robust preface addressed to the "blessed father." He vowed that he had to date "spoken only good and honorable words" concerning Leo, and offered to retract anything that might have betrayed "indiscretion and impiety." "I am the kind of person," he wrote in seeming earnest, "who would wish you all good things eternally."[14]

Luther was concerned, however, that the papal office had saddled Leo with a false sense of dignity. "You are a servant of servants" (*servus servorum*) within the church, Luther wrote to Leo, citing the classic title of the Bishop of Rome.[15] And as a "servant of God for others, and over others, and for the sake of others," you properly enjoy a "sublime dignity" of office.[16] But the "obsequious flatterers" and "pestilential fellows" of your papal court do not regard you as a humble servant. Instead, they treat you as "a vicar of Christ," as "a demigod [who] may command and require whatever you wish." They "pretend that you are lord of the world, allow no one to be considered a Christian unless he accepts your authority, and prate that you have power over heaven, hell and purgatory." Surely, you do not believe any of this, Luther wrote to Leo, tongue near cheek. Surely, you can see that "they err who ascribe to you alone the right of interpreting Scripture" and "who exalt you above a council and the church universal." "Perhaps I am being presumptuous" to address you so, Luther allowed at the end of his preface. But when a fellow Christian, even a pope, is exposed to such "dangerous" teachings and trappings, God commands that a fellow brother offer him biblical counsel, without regard for his "dignity or lack of dignity."[17]

In later pages of the *Freedom of a Christian* and in several other writings in that same crucial year of 1520, Luther took aim at other persons who were "puffed up because of their dignity."[18] He inveighed at greatest length against the lower clergy, who, in his view, used the "false power of fabricated sacraments" to "tyrannize the Christian conscience" and to "fleece the sheep" of Christendom.[19] He criticized jurists for spinning the thick tangle of special benefits, privileges, exemptions, and immunities that elevated the clergy above the laity and inoculated them from legal accountability to local magistrates.[20] He was not much kinder to princes, nobles, and merchants—those "harpies," as he later called them, "blinded by their arrogance" and trading on their office, pedigree, and wealth to lord it over the languishing commoner.[21] What all these pretentious folks fail to see, Luther wrote, is that "there is no basic difference in status . . . between laymen and priests, princes and bishops, religious and secular."[22] Before God all are equal.

Luther's *Freedom of a Christian* thus became, in effect, his *Dignitatis Humanae*—his bold new declaration on human nature and human freedom that described all Christians in his world regardless of their "dignity or lack of dignity," as conventionally defined. Pope and prince, noble and pauper, man and woman, slave and free—all persons in Christendom, Luther declared, share equally in a doubly paradoxical nature. First, each person is at once a saint and a sinner, righteous and reprobate, saved and lost—*simul iustus et peccator,* in Luther's signature phrase.[23] Second, each person is at once a free lord who is subject to no one and a dutiful servant who is subject to everyone. Only through these twin paradoxes, Luther wrote, can we "comprehend the lofty dignity of the Christian."[24]

Every Christian "has a twofold nature," Luther argued in expounding his doctrine of *simul iustus et peccator.* We are at once body and soul, flesh and spirit, sinner and saint, "outer man and inner man." These "two men in the same man contradict each other" and remain perennially at war.[25] On the one hand, as bodily creatures, we are born in sin and bound by sin. By our carnal natures, we are prone to lust and lasciviousness, evil and egoism, perversion and pathos of untold dimensions.[26] Even the best of persons, even the titans of virtue in the Bible—Abraham, David, Peter, and Paul—sin all the time.[27] In and of ourselves, we are totally depraved and deserving of eternal death. On the other hand, as spiritual creatures, we are reborn in faith and freed from sin. By our spiritual natures, we are prone to love and charity, goodness and sacrifice, virtue and peacefulness. Even the worst of persons, even the reprobate thief nailed on the next cross to Christ's, can be saved from sin. In spite of ourselves, we are totally redeemed and assured of eternal life.[28]

It is through faith and hope in the Word of God, Luther argued, that a person moves from sinner to saint, from bondage to freedom. This was the essence of Luther's doctrine of justification by faith alone. No human work of any sort—even worship, contemplation, meditation, charity, and other supposed meritorious conduct—can make a person just and righteous before God. For sin holds the person fast, and perverts his or her every work. "One thing, and only one thing, is necessary for Christian life, righteousness, and freedom," Luther declared. "That one thing is the most holy Word of God, the gospel of Christ."[29] To put one's faith in this Word, to accept its gracious promise of eternal salvation, is to claim one's freedom from sin and from its attendant threat of eternal damnation. And it is to join the communion of saints that begins imperfectly in this life and continues perfectly in the life to come.

A saint by faith remains a sinner by nature, Luther insisted, and the paradox of good and evil within the same person remains until death. But there is "a difference between sinners and sinners," Luther wrote. "There are some sinners who confess that they have sinned but do not long to be justified; instead, they give up hope and go on sinning so that when they die they despair, and while they live, they are enslaved to the world. There are other sinners who confess that they sin and have sinned, but they are sorry for this, hate themselves for it, long to be justified, and under groaning constantly pray to God for righteousness. This is the people of God," the saints who are saved, despite their sin.[30]

This brought Luther to a related paradox of human nature—that each Christian is at once a lord who is subject to no one and a priest who is servant to everyone. On the one hand, Luther argued, "every Christian is by faith so exalted above all things that, by virtue of a spiritual power, he is [a] lord."[31] As a redeemed saint, as an "inner man," a Christian is utterly free in his conscience, utterly free in his innermost being. He is like the greatest king on earth, who is above and beyond the power of everyone. No earthly authority—whether pope, prince, or parent—can impose "a single syllable of the law" upon him.[32] No earthly authority can intrude upon the sanctuary of his conscience, can endanger his assurance and comfort of eternal life. This is "the splendid privilege," the "inestimable power and liberty" that every Christian enjoys.[33]

On the other hand, Luther wrote, every Christian is a priest, who freely performs good works in service of his or her neighbor and in glorification of God.[34] "Christ has made it possible for us, provided we believe in him, to be not only his brethren, co-heirs, and fellow-kings, but also his fellow-priests," Luther wrote. And thus, in imitation of Christ, we freely serve our neighbors, offering instruction, charity, prayer, admonition, and sacrifice even to the point of death.[35] We abide by the law of God so far as we are able so that others may see our good work and be similarly impelled to seek God's grace. We freely discipline and drive ourselves to do as much good as we are able, not so that we may be saved but so that others may be served. "A man does not live for himself alone," Luther wrote, "he lives only for others."[36] The precise nature of our priestly service to others depends upon our gifts and upon the vocation in which God calls us to use them.[37] But we are all to serve freely and fully as God's priests.

"Who can then comprehend the lofty dignity of the Christian?" Luther wrote. "By virtue of his royal power he rules over all things, death, life, and sin." The person is entirely free from the necessity of doing good works and fully immune from the authority of anyone. But by virtue of "his priestly glory, he is omnipotent with God because he does the things which God asks and requires."[38] He devotes himself entirely to doing good works for his neighbor; he submits himself completely to the needs of others.

Such are the paradoxes of the Christian life in Luther's view. We are at once sinners and saints; we are at once lords and servants. We can do nothing good; we can do nothing but good. We are utterly free; we are everywhere bound. The more a person thinks himself a saint, the more sinful in fact he becomes. The more a person thinks herself a sinner, the more saintly she in fact becomes. The more a person acts like a lord, the more he is called to be a servant. The more a person acts as a servant, the more in fact she has become a lord. This is the paradoxical nature of human life. And this is the essence of human dignity.

Luther intended his *Freedom of a Christian* to be a universal statement for his world of Christendom—a summary of "the whole of the

Christian life in a brief form," as he put it in his preface to Leo.[39] He grounded his views in the Bible, liberally peppering his tract with all manner of biblical citations and quotations. He wove into his narrative several strong threads of argument pulled selectively from a number of Church Fathers and late medieval Christian mystics. He published his tract both in Latin and in simple German, seeking to reach both the scholar and the commoner alike. He wrote with a pastoral directness and emotional empathy, convinced that if he could point out the Jekyll and Hyde in everyone, his readers would find both ample humility and ample comfort. So convinced was Luther of the veracity and cogency of his views that he believed even the Jews, the one perennial sojourner in his world of Christendom, would convert en masse to the Gospel once they heard it in this simple form.[40] Though this latter aspiration proved fanciful, Luther's views on human dignity did command an impressive readership among Christians. *Freedom of a Christian* was a best-seller in its day—going through twelve printings in its first two years and five editions by 1524. It remained a perennial favorite of commentaries and sermons long after Luther's passing and well beyond the world of Lutheranism.[41] It is no small commentary on the enduring ecumenical efficacy of Luther's views of human nature, dignity, and freedom that they lie at the heart of the "Joint Declaration on the Doctrine of Justification," signed by Catholic and Evangelical leaders on October 31, 1999.

What all this elegant dialectic theology meant for the nature of freedom of the Christian in this world, Luther's little tract did not so clearly say. Luther did make clear that all Christians have the freedom and duty to follow the Bible conscientiously and to speak out against human ideas and institutions that conflict with the Bible. The Bible was for Luther the great equalizer of Christians—to the remarkable point of allowing Luther, a lowly Augustinian monk from an obscure German town, to address His Holiness Leo X as if he were the pope's equal. Luther also made clear that clergy and laity are fundamentally equal in dignity and responsibility before God. The traditional assumption that the clergy were superior to the laity and entitled to all manner of special privileges, immunities, and exemptions was anathema to Luther. Luther at once laicized the clergy and clericized the laity, treating the office of preaching and teaching as just one other vocation alongside many others that a conscientious Christian could properly and freely pursue.[42]

Luther's *Freedom of a Christian*, however, was no political manifesto on freedom. Spiritual freedom may well coexist with political bondage, Luther insisted. The spiritual equality of persons and vocations before God does not necessarily entail a social equality with all others.[43] Luther became doubly convinced of this discordance after witnessing the bloody Peasants' Revolt in Germany in 1525 and the growing numbers of radical egalitarian and antinomian experiments engineered out of his favorite theological doctrines of the priesthood of all believers and justification by faith alone. In the course of the next two decades, Luther defended with increasing stridency traditional social, economic, political, and ecclesiastical hierarchies as a necessary feature of this earthly life.

Luther came to defend this disparity between the spiritual and temporal dimensions of human freedom, dignity, and status with his doctrine of the two kingdoms. God has ordained two kingdoms or realms in which humanity is destined to live, Luther argued: the earthly or political kingdom and the heavenly or spiritual kingdom. The earthly kingdom is the realm of creation, of natural and civic life, where a person operates primarily by reason, law, and passion. The heavenly kingdom is the realm of redemption, of spiritual and eternal life, where a person operates primarily by faith, hope, and charity. These two kingdoms embrace parallel forms of righteousness and justice, truth and knowledge, but they remain separate and distinct. The earthly kingdom is distorted by sin and governed by the law. The heavenly kingdom is renewed by grace and guided by the Gospel. A Christian is a citizen of both kingdoms at once and invariably comes under the distinctive jurisdiction of each kingdom. As a heavenly citizen, the Christian remains free in his conscience, called to live fully by the light of the Word of God. But as an earthly citizen, the Christian is bound by law and called to obey the structures and strictures of ecclesiastical, political, and parental authority, even if they are sometimes hard and abusive.

Protestant Instincts about Human Dignity and Freedom Today

Nearly half a millennium after its publication, Luther's *Freedom of a Christian* still shapes many Protestants' instincts about human dignity and human freedom. First, Luther's doctrine of *simul iustus et peccator* renders many Protestants instinctively skeptical about too optimistic a view of human nature and too easy a conflation of human dignity and human sanctity. Such views take too little account of the radicality of human sin and the necessity of divine grace. They give too little credibility to the inherent human need for discipline and order, accountability and judgment. They give too little credence to the perennial interplay of the civil, theological, and pedagogical uses of law, to the perpetual demand to balance deterrence, retribution, and reformation in discharging authority within the home, church, state, and other associations. They give too little insight into the necessity for safeguarding every office of authority from abuse and misuse. A theory of human dignity that fails to take into account the combined depravity and sanctity of the human person is theologically and politically deficient, if not dangerous.

This cardinal insight into the twofold nature of humanity was hardly unique to Martin Luther and is readily amenable to many other formulations. Luther's formula of *simul iustus et peccator* was a crisp Christian distillation of a universal insight about human nature that can be traced to the earliest Greek and Hebrew sources of the West. The gripping tragedies of Homer, Hesiod, and Pindar are nothing if not chronicles of the perennial dialectic of good and evil, virtue and vice, hero and villain in the ancient Greek world. The very first chapters of the Hebrew Bible paint pictures of these same two human natures, now with Yahweh's imprint on them. The more familiar picture is that of Adam and Eve, who were created equally in the image of God and vested with a natural right and duty to perpetuate life, to cultivate property, to dress and keep the creation (Gen. 1:26–30; 2:7, 15–23). The less familiar picture is that of their first child Cain, who murdered his brother Abel and was called into judgment by God and condemned for his sin. Yet "God put a mark on Cain," Genesis reads, both to protect him in his life, and to show that he remained a child of God despite the enormity of his sin (Gen. 4:1–16).[44] One message of this ancient Hebrew text is that we are not only the beloved children of Adam and Eve, who bear the image of God, with all the divine perquisites and privileges of Paradise. We are also the sinful siblings of Cain, who bear the mark of God, with its ominous assurance both that we shall be called into divine judgment for what we have done and that there is forgiveness even for the gravest of sins we have committed.

Luther believed that it is only through faith and hope in Christ that we can ultimately be assured of divine forgiveness and eternal salvation. He further believed that it was only through a life of biblical meditation, prayer, worship, charity, and sacramental living that a person could hold his or her depravity in check and aspire to greater sanctity. I believe that, too, as do many Christians today. But this is not to say that, in this life, Christians have the only insights into the twofold nature of humanity, and the only effective means of balancing the realities of human depravity and the aspirations for human sanctity. Any religious tradition that takes seriously the Jekyll and Hyde in all of us has its own understanding of ultimate reconciliation of these two natures, and its own methods of balancing them in this life. And who are we Christians to say how God will ultimately judge these?

Luther also believed that the ominous assurance of the judgment of God is ultimately a source of comfort not of fear. The first sinners in the Bible—Adam, Eve, and Cain—were given divine due process: They were confronted with the evidence, asked to defend themselves, given a chance to repent, spared the ultimate sanction of death, and then assured of a second trial on the Day of Judgment, with appointed divine counsel—Christ himself, our self-appointed "advocate before the Father" (1 John 2:1). The only time that God deliberately withheld divine due process was in the capital trial of His Son—and that was the only time it was and has been necessary. The political implications of this are very simple: If God gives due process in judging us, we should give due process in judging others. If God's tribunals feature at least basic rules of procedure, evidence, representation, and advocacy, human tribunals should feature at least the same. The demand for due process is a deep human instinct, and it has driven Protestants over the centuries, along with many others before and with them, to be strident advocates for procedural rights.

Second, Luther's doctrine of the lordship and priesthood of all believers renders many Protestants instinctively jealous about liberty and equality—but on their own quite distinct theological terms. In the modern liberal tradition, liberty and equality are generally defended on grounds of popular sovereignty and inalienable rights. The American Declaration of Independence (1776) proclaimed it a "self-evident truth" "that all men are created equal [and] . . . are endowed with certain unalienable rights." The Universal Declaration of Human Rights (1948) proclaimed "[t]hat all men are born free and equal in rights and dignity." Protestants can resonate more with the norms of liberty and equality in these documents than with the theories of popular sovereignty and inalienable rights that generally undergird them.

The heart of the Protestant theory of liberty is that we are all lords on this earth. We are utterly free in the sanctuary of our conscience, entirely unencumbered in our relationship with God. We enjoy a sovereign immunity from any human structures and strictures, even those of the church when they seek to impose upon this divine freedom. Such talk of "sovereign immunity" sounds something like modern liberal notions of "popular sovereignty." And such talk of "lordship" sounds something like the democratic right to "self-rule." Protestants have thus long found ready allies in liberals and others who advocate liberty of conscience and democratic freedoms on these grounds. But, when theologically pressed, many Protestants will defend liberty of conscience not because of their own popular sovereignty, but because of the absolute sovereignty of God, whose relationship with his children cannot be trespassed. Many Protestants will defend certain inalienable rights, like freedom of conscience, not in the interest of preserving their personal privacy, but in the interest of discharging their divine duties.

The heart of the Protestant theory of equality is that we are all priests before God. "You are a chosen race, a royal priesthood, a holy nation, God's own people" (1 Pet. 2:9; cf. Rev. 5:10; and Rev. 20:6). Among you, "[t]here is neither Jew nor Greek, there is neither slave nor free, there is neither male nor female; for you are all one in Christ Jesus" (Gal. 3:28; cf. Col. 3:10–11; Eph. 2:14–15). These and many other biblical passages, which Luther highlighted and glossed repeatedly, have long inspired a reflexive egalitarian impulse in Protestants. All are equal before God. All are priests that must serve their neighbors. All have vocations that count. All have gifts to be included. This common calling of all to be priests transcends differences of culture, economy, gender, and more.

Such teachings have led a few Protestant groups over the centuries to experiment with intensely communitarian states of nature where life is gracious, lovely, and long. Most Protestant groups, however, view life in such states of nature as brutish, nasty, and short, for sin invariably perverts them. Structures and strictures of law and authority are necessary and useful, most Protestants believe. But such structures need to be as open, egalitarian, and democratic as possible. Hierarchy is a danger to be indulged only so far as necessary. To be sure, Protestants over the centuries have often defied these founding ideals, and have earnestly partaken of all manner of elitism, chauvinism, racism, anti-semitism, tyranny, patriarchy, slavery, apartheid, and more. And they have sometimes engaged in outrageous hypocrisy and casuistry to defend such shameful pathos. But an instinct for egalitarianism—for embracing all persons equally, for treating all vocations respectfully, for arranging all associations horizontally, for leveling the life of the earthly kingdom so none is obstructed in access to God—is a Lutheran gene in the theo-logical genetic code of Protestantism.

Third and finally, Luther's notion that a person is at once free and bound by the law has powerful implications for our modern under-standing of human rights. For Luther, the Christian is free in order to follow the commandments of the faith—or, in more familiar and gen-eral modern parlance, a person has rights in order to discharge duties. Freedoms and commandments, rights and duties belong together in Luther's formulation. To speak of one without the other is ultimately destructive. Rights without duties to guide them quickly become claims of self-indulgence. Duties without rights to exercise them quickly become sources of deep guilt.

Protestants have thus long translated the moral duties set out in the Decalogue into reciprocal rights. The First Table of the Decalogue pre-scribes duties of love that each person owes to God—to honor God and God's name, to observe the Sabbath day of rest and holy worship, to avoid false gods and false swearing. The Second Table prescribes duties of love that each person owes to neighbors—to honor one's parents and other authorities, not to kill, not to commit adultery, not to steal, not to bear false witness, not to covet. Church, state, and family alike are re-sponsible for the communication and enforcement of these cardinal moral duties, Protestants have long argued. But it is also the responsi-bility of each person to ensure that he and his neighbors discharge these moral duties. This is one important impetus for Protestants to translate duties into rights. A person's duties toward God can be cast as the rights of religion: the right to honor God and God's name, the right to rest and worship on one's Sabbath, the right to be free from false gods and false oaths. Each person's duties toward a neighbor, in turn, can be cast as a neighbor's right to have that duty discharged. One person's duties not to kill, to commit adultery, to steal, or to bear false witness thus give rise to another person's rights to life, property, fidelity, and reputation. For a person to insist upon vindication of these latter rights is not necessarily to act out of self-love. It is also to act out of neighborly love. To claim one's own right is in part a charitable act to induce one's neighbor to discharge his or her divinely ordained duty.

The great American jurist Grant Gilmore once wrote: "The better the society the less law there will be. In Heaven, there will be no law, and the lion will lie down with the lamb. In Hell, there will be nothing but law, and due process will be meticulously observed."[45] This is a rather common Protestant sentiment, which Luther did much to propound in some of his early writings. But a Protestant, faithful to Luther's most enduring insights, might properly reach the exact opposite projection. In Heaven, there will be pure law, and thus the lamb will lie down with the lion. In Hell, there will be no law, and thus all will devour each other eternally. Heaven will exalt due process, and each will always receive what's due. Hell will exalt pure caprice, and no one will ever know what's coming.

Notes

Portions of this essay are drawn from my *Law and Protestantism: The Legal Teachings of the Lutheran Reformation* (Cambridge and New York: Cambridge University Press, 2002). I wish to thank Don Browning, Timothy P. Jackson, Robert Kraynak, and Glenn Tinder for their very helpful comments on an earlier draft of this essay. I would like to thank Jeffrey Hammond and Penelope Brady for their research assistance.

1. Reprinted in Walter M. Abbott and J. Gallagher, eds., *The Documents of Vatican II* (New York: Herder & Herder, 1966), 675.

2. The term "ur-principle" is from Louis Henkin et al., *Human Rights* (New York: Foundation Press, 1999), 80.

3. Reprinted in Ian Brownlie, ed., *Basic Documents on Human Rights,* 3d ed. (Oxford: Oxford University Press, 1992), 21.

4. *Pacem in Terris* (1963), par. 9, reprinted in Joseph Gremillion, ed., *The Gospel of Peace and Justice: Catholic Social Teaching since Pope John* (Maryknoll, N.Y.: Orbis Books, 1976), 201, 203.

5. See ibid.; and *Dignitatis Humanae* (1965), in *Documents of Vatican II,* 675.

6. See, e.g., Allen O. Miller, ed., *A Christian Declaration on Human Rights* (Grand Rapids: Wm. Eerdmans, 1977) (a Calvinist statement, with full endorsement of the concept of human dignity); Lutheran World Federation, *Theological Perspectives on Human Rights* (Geneva, 1977) (a Lutheran document that largely eschews the concept of human dignity); *Human Rights and Christian Responsibility*, 3 vols. (Geneva: World Council of Churches, 1975) (ecumenical statements with only passing references to human dignity). See detailed analysis in Wolfgang Huber and Heinz Eduard Tödt, *Menschenrechte: Perspektiven einer menschlichen Welt* (Stuttgart: Kreuz Verlag, 1977); Wolfgang Vögele, *Menschenwürde zwischen Recht und Theologie: Begründungen von Menschenrechte in der Perspektive öffentlicher Theologie* (Gütersloh: Chr. Kaiser, 2001).

7. See the preambles to both documents in *Basic Documents on Human Rights*, 114, 125.

8. International Convention on the Elimination of all Forms of Racial Discrimination (1969), preface, in *Basic Documents on Human Rights*, 148. See comparable language in International Convention on Suppression and Punishment of the Crime of Apartheid (1973), in ibid., 162; Convention on the Elimination of All Forms of Discrimination against Women (1979), in ibid., 169.

9. See, e.g., sources and discussion in Carl Wellmann, *The Proliferation of Rights: Moral Progress or Empty Rhetoric* (Boulder/Oxford: Westview Press, 1999).

10. See, e.g., sources and discussion in John Witte, Jr., and Johan D. van der Vyver, eds., *Religious Human Rights in Global Perspective*, 2 vols. (The Hague/London/Boston: Martinus Nijhoff, 1996).

11. See, e.g., David Novak, *Covenantal Rights* (Princeton: Princeton University Press, 2001); Abdullahi Ahmed An-Na'im, *Toward an Islamic Revolution: Civil Liberties, Human Rights, and International Law* (Syracuse: Syracuse University Press, 1990); Wm. Theodore de Bary and Tu Weiming, eds., *Confucianism and Human Rights* (New York: Columbia University Press, 1998); Irene Bloom, J. Paul Martin, and Wayne L. Proudfoot, eds., *Religious Diversity and Human Rights* (New York: Columbia University Press, 1996).

12. See, e.g., Herschel Baker, *The Image of Man: A Study of the Idea of Human Dignity in Classical Antiquity, the Middle Ages, and the Renaissance* (New York: Harper & Bros., 1961); Charles Trinkaus, *"In Our Image and Likeness": Humanity and Divinity in Italian Humanist Thought*, 2 vols. (London and Chicago: University of Chicago Press, 1970); Jürgen Moltmann, *On Human Dignity, Political Theology and Ethics*, trans. M. Douglas Meeks (Philadelphia: Fortress Press, 1984).

13. *De Libertate Christiana* (1520), in *D. Martin Luthers Werke: Kritische Gesamtausgabe* (Weimar, 1883–), 7:49–73 [hereafter WA], translated in Jaroslav Pelikan et al., eds., *Luther's Works* (Philadelphia: Muhlenberg Press, 1955–),

31:327–377 [hereafter LW]. A shorter German edition, *Die Freiheit eines Christen-menschen*, appears in WA 7:20–38.

14. LW 31:334–36.

15. LW 31:341.

16. LW 31:341, 342. The quote is from *Luther: Lectures on Romans* [1515–1516], trans. Wilhelm Pauck (Philadelphia: Westminster Press, 1961), 8. Many of the teachings from these lectures are repeated in Luther's *Freedom of a Christian*.

17. LW 31:341–42. See similar sentiments in Luther's *Address to the Christian Nobility of the German Nation Concerning the Reform of the Christian Estate* (1520), LW 44:123–217, at 136.

18. Quotation is from Luther's *Lectures on Genesis*, 38–44 (1544), LW 7:182.

19. See esp. LW 44:126–55; *The Babylonian Captivity of the Church* (1520), LW 36:11–126; *Treatise on Good Works* (1520), LW 44:21–114, at 87–94, with expansion in *The Keys* (1530), LW 40:321–70. In LW 44:158, Luther recommended that a new imperial law be passed against papal appointments of clergy so that "no confirmation of any dignity whatsoever shall henceforth be secured from Rome." In LW 44:129 and LW 36:117, Luther attacked the notion that the clergy were special because of the "indelible mark" of their ordination, terming this "a laughingstock."

20. LW 44:157ff., 202ff.

21. LW 7:182ff.; LW 44:203ff. See also Luther's fuller statement in *Temporal Authority: To What Extent It Should Be Obeyed* (1523), in LW 45:75–129.

22. LW 44:129.

23. LW 31:344–47, 358–61. The theme recurs repeatedly in Luther's later writings. See, e.g., LW 12:328, 27:230ff., 32:173; WA 39/1:21, 492, 552.

24. LW 31:355.

25. LW 31:344.

26. LW 31:344, 358–61; see also LW 25:120–30, 204–13.

27. See, e.g., LW 19:47–48, LW 23:146.

28. LW 31:344–54, 368–77.

29. LW 31:345.

30. *Lectures on Romans*, 120. See also LW 23:146; LW 12:328–30; LW 8:9–12.

31. LW 31:354.

32. LW 36:70, echoing LW 31:344–46.

33. LW 31:355–58.

34. LW 31:355–56. Luther returned to this theme repeatedly in his later writings. See, e.g., LW 36:112–16, 138–40; LW 40:21–23; LW 13:152, and esp. the long diatribe in LW 39:137–224.

35. LW 31:355; see also LW 36:241.

36. LW 31:364–65; see also LW 51:86–87.

37. LW 38:188; LW 28:171–72.

38. LW 31:355; see also LW 17:209ff.

39. LW 31:343.

40. See *That Jesus Christ Was Born a Jew* (1523), in LW 45:129. See further Steven E. Ozment, *Protestants: The Birth of a Revolution* (New York: Doubleday, 1992), 1; idem, "Martin Luther on Religious Liberty," in Noel B. Reynolds and W. Cole Durham, Jr., eds., *Religious Liberty in Western Thought* (Atlanta: Scholars Press, 1996), 75.

41. Mark U. Edwards, Jr., *Printing, Propaganda, and Martin Luther* (Berkeley, Calif.: University of California Press, 1981), 39, 64, 100–101.

42. See further *Concerning the Ministry* (1523), in LW 40:21ff.

43. LW 31:354–56, 364–65.

44. This is but one of numerous interpretations of the story of Cain and Abel. For alternatives, see Ruth Mellinkoff, *The Mark of Cain* (Berkeley: University of California Press, 1981); Claus Westermann, *Genesis 1–11: A Commentary,* repr. ed. (Minneapolis: Augsburg Publishing House, 1990).

45. Grant Gilmore, *The Ages of American Law* (Chicago: University of Chicago Press, 1977), 110–11.

CHAPTER FIVE

A House Divided, Again: Sanctity vs. Dignity in the Induced Death Debates

TIMOTHY P. JACKSON

"A house divided against itself cannot stand."
—Abraham Lincoln, echoing Mark 3:25

The philosophy of liberal democracy ascendant in the West since the eighteenth century—with its accent on civil equality, individual liberty, and the rule of law—has arguably been the most effective political defender of the dignity of persons ever devised. The breakdown of class divisions, the protection of freedom of conscience, the enumeration of universal human rights, the abolition of slavery, the progressive liberation of women, all stand among the truly remarkable ethical achievements of the last three centuries. Much remains to be done even within the narrow confines of politics, of course; prejudices based on race, class, gender, ethnicity, and sexual orientation continue to divide us into intolerant and sometimes warring camps. But any account of our situation that denies the advances of the last three hundred years forgets who most of us are or aspire to be. That said, my central thesis in this essay is that the emphasis on "personal dignity" that is one of the chief Western glories now threatens to subvert our moral lives.

For some time now, our most perceptive social critics have been warning us that "freedom" is becoming an excuse for selfishness toward those who are unfree and "reason" an occasion for cruelty toward those judged irrational or nonrational.[1] We are often so concerned to respect the choices of autonomous agents that we not only become blind to other treasures but also neglect the context and necessary conditions for agency itself. There are many possible explanations for this degradation: misguided neutrality claimed by the state sometimes caused by religious dogmatism or would-be tolerance of divergent viewpoints leading to unhistorical separations of "religion" from "politics." But it is increasingly clear at the beginning of the twenty-first century that the "enlightened" safeguarding of existing persons threatens the genesis of personhood itself. Valorization of "the personal" (especially rational individuality) menaces a range of impersonal yet indispensable values (from the environment to future generations).

Dignity has become increasingly forgetful of its origin in sanctity, respect for persons unmindful of the fact that persons only emerge out of impersonal needs and potentials that are addressed by grace, whether human or divine. Secular thinkers may speak of the gratuitious care of parents for children, while theists refer to the providence of God sustaining the world, but these are commonly thought to be "private" rather than "public" concerns. In turn, the rational calculation of justice (what persons are due by right based on self-conscious interest) has been largely alienated from both the loving creation and the emotional appreciation of value (what is inherently good though often unselfconscious).

Thus I contrast in this essay what I call "an ethic of pure dignity" with a moral vision that attends to both dignity and sanctity. By "pure dignity" I mean an exclusive emphasis on self-conscious autonomy, the ability to form rational intentions and execute independent decisions over time, as the criterion for valuable (personal) identity. Such an emphasis tends to exalt reason and volition to the exclusion of such "embodied" faculties as passion, hunger, laughter, forgiveness, and growth. A more holistic and historical ethic, on the other hand, will also take sanctity into account. As I define the term, "sanctity" refers to the impersonal (i.e., humanly shared) needs and potentials that are antecedent to any calculable merit or achievement. In opposition to the radical cognitivism and voluntarism of pure dignity, sanctity encompasses such elements of "noncognitive well-being"[2] as the capacity to feel joy, the need to receive care, and the potential to be loved.

The word "sanctity" often has religious overtones, but it need not be understood in explicitly theistic terms, e.g., as a creation of the biblical God. (Even some atheists believe in the "sanctity" of human life.) My own views are Christian, but I mean the above definition to leave open the question of the source of our shared needs and potentials; a benevolent deity, an orderly nature, or a purely contingent evolution might be pointed to—though perhaps not with equal plausibility. In so far as it points to goods that are not intentionally constructed or individually earned by human beings, at any rate, "sanctity" connotes a gracious giftedness. It gestures toward those forces larger than ourselves, found rather than made, by which we live. If dignity calls forth respect or admiration for some personal exploit, then sanctity evokes a more amorphous awe and wonder.

One might base observations about the "triumph" of dignity on any number of ethical literatures, but I want to focus on aspects of the recent debates around induced death: abortion and euthanasia. In a 1997 piece entitled "Assisted Suicide: The Philosophers' Brief,"[3] several prominent American philosophers weighed in favoring a right to die, including a right to practitioner-assisted suicide (PAS). The signers (*amici curiae*) were Ronald Dworkin, Thomas Nagel, Robert Nozick, John Rawls, Thomas Scanlon, and Judith Jarvis Thomson. In his 1994 book, *Rethinking Life and Death,* the Australian utilitarian Peter Singer also endorsed forms of euthanasia, again including PAS. The subtitle of Singer's text was "The Collapse of Our Traditional Ethics"—"traditional ethics" meaning a commitment to the sanctity of all human life. If one couples "The Philosophers' Brief" and *Rethinking Life and Death* with the 1994 edition of Thomas Beauchamp and James Childress's influential *Principles of Biomedical Ethics,* a surprising convergence of philosophical opinion appears. For Beauchamp and Childress now defend active euthanasia under certain circumstances as well.[4]

Indeed, concerning euthanasia a sea change in America in the 1990s seems comparable to abortion-related developments in the late 1960s and early 1970s. The covert practice of active euthanasia,[5] including PAS, has been underway for some time,[6] even as forms of abortion were available long before *Roe v. Wade* (1973). But public opinion and legal policy are now shifting explicitly to permit what was once officially prohibited. The recent Oregon referendum upholding that state's Death with Dignity Act may well provide the sort of historic marker around the end of life that *Roe v. Wade* now provides around the beginning of life. Still, the reasons for the emerging policy consensus remain complicated, if not contradictory;[7] as with abortion, euthanasia rationales vary, and it is unclear what types of reasons can legitimately be introduced into civic speech. In spite of the appearance of an increasingly united front, deep divisions remain. On matters of life and death, the American house is deeply divided, with some views not merely opposed but ruled out of court by "liberal" positions.

Specifically, I aim to do four things here: (1) to set abortion and euthanasia discussions against the general background of the relation between human sanctity and personal dignity; (2) to note, more specifically, how both Dworkin and Singer tend to exclude sanctity (a.k.a. "religious") considerations from public debate a priori; (3) to draw out what is, nevertheless, a significant difference between them; and (4) to gesture toward an alternative to both positions that defends, morally and legally, the sanctity of human life. The alternative is indebted to Simone Weil and is Christian in inspiration, though it is not the only possible Christian position.

My thesis is that neither deontological theories of justice nor utilitarian accounts of value have a presumptive claim on a democratic polis. The sanctity of human life is as publicly defensible by a prophetic liberalism as the dignity of persons is by any secular liberalism. More emphatically, neither the separation of value from legally enforceable interest-based rights (Dworkin) nor the identification of value preeminently, if not exclusively, with self-conscious bearers of interests (Singer) provides a viable basis for a just society. In neglecting to support human life in its most vulnerable stages, germinal and geriatric, neither school can nurture and sustain the very persons it would protect.

Christian convictions about sanctity will quite possibly lose out in the twenty-first-century debates concerning life and death, but they ought not to be excluded from public discourse as such. Indeed, if theological beliefs about sanctity are judged illegitimate by the new "liberal" culture, so must all substantive accounts (religious or secular) of human needs and potentials. Excluding such accounts produces an artificial policy convergence that masks two profound distinctions, however: that between sanctity and dignity in the moral life and that between deontology and utility in moral philosophy. If the social divisions that grow up around these distinctions are not acknowledged and democratically adjudicated, civil war is one possible result. If, to echo Lincoln, a house divided against itself (half slave and half free) cannot continue to stand, then one so divided as to preclude recognition of what it is (religious and secular, impersonal and personal) may have already fallen.

Dignity and Sanctity

On one common reading, "dignity" refers to a basic faculty; it denotes the bare capacity for intelligent free choice[8] shared equally by all non-damaged persons. One's rational freedom may be misused, but the simple possession of it is the ground of respect. Kant, for instance, held that all persons are to be treated as ends, and not as means only, because they are capable of acting autonomously—i.e., according to imperatives they willingly give to themselves. On another reading, in contrast, "dignity" is a term of achievement; it requires that actual choices be meritorious or at least morally responsible. Here respect awaits some historical performance that claims our special acknowledgement; only a limited number of individuals (e.g., the noble) possess personal dignity and the rights that go along with it. An ethic emphasizing dignity as something given will tend, naturally, to equality; one in which dignity is something achieved, to hierarchy.

Both of these senses of "dignity" are at work in liberal political contexts, and it is important to appreciate the differences between them. For present purposes, however, a fundamental similarity is most germane. On both readings, dignity is a function of the freedom of self-conscious agents, their ability to choose intentionally, or their having chosen rightly or virtuously. Indeed, even if dignity is taken to stem from simple rational agency, rather than actual excellent choices, it still requires that a threshold of cognitive maturation be reached. Even the first sense of "dignity" demands, after all, a kind of achievement—namely, that one has passed one's spiritual nonage and acquired a fairly robust self-awareness. Only subjects who are aware of themselves as abiding rational agents are "persons," properly so-called, on this view.

A liberal society may champion dignity, then, both by clearing space de jure for all persons to act freely and by adjudicating the interest claims that arise from de facto free actions across time. But immediately three groups of humans become "problematized" by this approach. Note that nothing has been said so far about human lives that are pre-personal (the very young), post-personal (the senile), or never-personal (the profoundly retarded). Indeed, nothing substantive can be said if dignity is the sole concern of liberal reflection. Both clearing space for personal freedom (e.g., protection of the individual from sacrifice to general utility) and adjudicating personal claims (e.g., enforcement of valid contracts) are indispensable matters of justice. A problem arises, however, when justice, defined as giving extant persons what their rational dignity demands, is taken to be the overriding (if not the only) political virtue. Such an elevation of justice ignores two crucial facts: (1) there are other values than personhood, even within the political sphere, and (2) personhood itself does not just happen but must be cultivated historically. Various aesthetic and ecological goods, as well as both fetal and senile human beings, are nonpersonal yet politically salient. And the dignity associated with autonomous agency—whether defined as a basic capacity or a contingent performance—depends on a sanctity given loving attention rather than mere procedural justice.

"Sanctity" is sometimes used as if synonymous with "dignity," to be sure; some authors, especially those writing within the Judeo-Christian tradition, use both terms to affirm the incalculable worth of all human beings.[9] But the two terms have increasingly floated free of one another in secular literature. As noted, dignity is now frequently associated with the present faculty of autonomy and/or the expressed desires of autonomous persons; sanctity, on the other hand, is traditionally a matter of the essential potentials and vital needs of all human lives. Sanctity, what the Christian tradition calls "being made in the Image of God," is most fundamentally the ability to give or receive loving care (*agape*). As such, sanctity is both pre- and post-personal, something coextensive with humanity itself. Because it makes sense to talk of non-voluntary development and noncognitive well-being, fetuses, babes in arms, the frail elderly, as well as the permanently demented may all be said to benefit from loving care. Although they are not "rational persons," in the technical sense described above, these human beings have needs and capabilities that can be addressed constructively by others and/or by God. They can be served as fellow creatures, and this ser-

vice redounds to both their and others' good. They possess a sanctity
to be honored, in short, even if not an achieved dignity to be respected.

If justice looks to the temporal claims of self-aware actors, and thus
is centrally appreciative of worth and agency, love attends to the enduring liabilities and prospects of embodied souls and thus is chiefly productive of worth and agency.[10] Sanctity precedes dignity, in that we are
all vulnerable and dependent human lives before (and possibly after) we
are reflective and autonomous persons; and love precedes justice, in that
if impersonal human lives are not cared for, there will be no earthly persons with rational wills to be respected. Sanctity and dignity are not
opposed, any more than love and justice, but you cannot have the latter
of either pair without the former.[11] More concretely, an ethic of "pure
dignity" in which autonomy alone has a claim on us will see little or
no reason to flinch from infanticide (as well as elective abortion) or from
nonvoluntary euthanasia (as well as assisted suicide); therefore, such an
ethic must call into question its own long-term viability.

The fact that respecting personal entitlement cannot be separated
from honoring human value is made evident by the problems presented
by Ronald Dworkin and Peter Singer, and I turn now to their illustrative work.

Dworkin and Singer: Striking Similarities

The first similarity to note between Dworkin and Singer is an emphasis on personal liberty and control: for them, individual freedom means,
primarily, freedom from constraint by others (negative freedom). In his
introduction to "The Philosophers' Brief," Dworkin appeals to

> a very general moral and constitutional principle—that every com-
> petent person has the right to make momentous personal decisions
> which invoke fundamental religious or philosophical convictions
> about life's value for himself. (41)

The brief itself argues that "respect for fundamental principles of liberty and justice, as well as for the American Constitutional tradition,
requires that the decisions of the Courts of Appeals [allowing the right
to assisted suicide] be affirmed" (43).

For his part, Singer holds that "[t]he desire among citizens of modern democracies for control over how they die is growing" and that the desire for such control "marks a sharp turning away from the sanctity of life ethic."[12] This turning, he maintains,

> will not be satisfied by the concessions to patient autonomy within the framework of that [the sanctity of life] ethic—a right to refuse "extraordinary means" of medical treatment, or to employ drugs like morphine that are "intended" to relieve pain, but have the "unintended but foreseen side-effect" of shortening life.[13]

The second similarity between Dworkin and Singer is a rejection of both the active/passive euthanasia distinction and the principle of double effect. In the case of Singer, it is easy to see how the rejection follows from his consequentialism. If the valuable end is release from personal suffering, then it does not matter how it is brought about, actively or passively; correlatively, double effect is otiose, in Singer's utilitarian view, since the net effect is the same, regardless of motive or means: a dead patient.

It is somewhat harder to see why leading deontologists might reject the distinction and principle in question, until one realizes that Dworkin, for instance, defines (legal) justice in terms of the adjudication of individual interests. He argues that neither the courts nor the Constitution should pronounce on questions of value, including the value and meaning of human life. Instead, they should be concerned only with the upholding of the rights of extant persons, especially the right to control their own lives without governmental coercion. As "The Philosophers' Brief" puts it, in discussing the Washington and New York cases then before the United States Supreme Court:

> These cases do not invite or require the Court to make moral, ethical, or religious judgments about how people should approach or control their death or about when it is ethically appropriate to hasten one's own death or to ask others for help in doing so. On the contrary, they ask the Court to recognize that individuals have a constitutionally protected interest in making those grave judgments for themselves, free from the imposition of any religious or philosophical orthodoxy by court or legislature. . . .

> Denying [the] opportunity [for physician assisted suicide] to
> terminally ill patients who are in agonizing pain or otherwise
> doomed to an existence they regard as intolerable could only be jus-
> tified on the basis of a religious or ethical conviction about the value
> or meaning of life itself. Our Constitution forbids government to
> impose such convictions on its citizens. (43)

In short, Dworkin et al. draw a sharp contrast between questions of
value/the good (such as the sanctity of life) and questions of justice/the
right (such as the fair adjudication of the liberty interests of persons).
They then go on to argue that legal sanctions should only be applied
in the latter context. The active/passive euthanasia distinction and the
principle of double effect simply do not get off the ground when a competent person wishes to die, for instance, because these notions depend
on a substantive conception of the value or meaning of human agency
that is overridden by an expression of agency itself. Dignity always
trumps in politics, on this analysis.

A third similarity between Dworkin and Singer is that they define
personhood in terms of the ability to be self-aware across time, to form
plans and intentions, to make autonomous choices, etc.[14] This convergence is the most profound, in that it tends to move both men (and it
is not insignificant that they are men) to glorify mind and will to the disregard of other human qualities. Self-awareness and self-control are the
sine qua non; without these, one is not a person with full legal standing.

A Key Difference

Despite the similarities outlined between Dworkin and Singer, a key
difference remains. In *Life's Dominion,* for instance, Dworkin acknowledges the intrinsic worth of various nonpersonal goods, including the
sanctity of human life, even when that life is fetal.[15] There is an important place for a wide range of judgments of intrinsic value in a well-
lived life (e.g., aesthetic evaluations of works of art), according to
Dworkin, but he nonetheless insists that the steel of the law must
remain neutral in this regard. Dworkin may believe in human sanctity,
but this is not the law's business. To repeat, the law adjudicates the
interest-based rights of existing persons only, remaining agnostic about
controversial axiological issues, however morally important.

Singer, in contrast, more explicitly allows both medicine and law to make quality of life judgments.[16] Or, better, he seems to leave far less room for intrinsic value outside of or beyond personal value—i.e., outside of or beyond the worth of persons able to form rational intentions—than does Dworkin. Singer does grant some moral significance to consciousness, in addition to self-consciousness, in the sense that he holds that sentient beings with the ability to feel pleasure and the desire to avoid pain ought not to be tormented.[17] But only autonomous persons have an inherent right to life, on his view. According to Singer, not all human life has a claim on us, whether one calls this "sanctity" or "dignity"; some human life is of insufficient quality or desirability to be worthy of respect and protection. Those who are in a persistently vegetative state, for example, are alive but effectively worthless. Singer goes so far as to remark that "life without consciousness is of no worth at all,"[18] so the persistently vegetative are candidates for nonvoluntary active euthanasia. In addition, it follows from Singer's cognitivist criteria that "newborn infants, especially if unwanted, are not yet full members of the moral community."[19]

Indeed, both fetuses and one-month-old babies may be directly and legally killed as nonpersons, according to Singer, subject to the autonomous choices of their parents. As Singer puts it, "in the case of infanticide, it is our culture that has something to learn from others, especially now that we, like them, are in a situation where we must limit family size"; thus "a period of twenty-eight days after birth might be allowed before an infant is accepted as having the same right to life as others."[20] Because fetuses and newborns have no awareness of themselves as existing over time, they are nonpersons, with at most a tenuous claim to life that can be trumped by the desires of adults. This goes for all fetuses and newborns, not merely disabled ones, since Singer denies real standing to any being without intentionality and self-awareness; as he puts it, "only a person has a right to life."[21] Like lower animals, unself-conscious human infants are interchangeable and can be killed at adult discretion so long as this is done mercifully, without causing suffering.[22] Dolphins, chimpanzees, and other higher mammals, on the other hand, are persons in Singer's sense; thus, they may not be killed or injured upon human demand. To think otherwise is speciesist, in his estimation.

A Christian Response

How might a Christian ethicist respond to Dworkin and Singer?

There are three related steps in Dworkin's argument, each of which is implausible by orthodox Christian lights: (1) the separation of intrinsic value from social justice, (2) the equation of social justice exclusively with the protection of rights, and (3) the reduction of rights to matters of self-conscious personal interest. With regard to step (1), Dworkin fails to see that some values are so foundational to justice itself that they may be given legal defense. Human life, even in its nascent stages, is one of these values. If both social and natural environments are not protected sufficiently to make future generations possible, then no form of justice as the balancing of personal interests will be possible. With regard to step (2), having intrinsic value does not directly entail having rights that must be justly balanced; as Dworkin points out, we think of a beautiful painting or sculpture as valuable (perhaps even sacred), without ascribing rights to it. But in the case of early human lives, part of their intrinsic worth is the fact that they will naturally grow into beings with interests and therefore rights, even as those rights will develop across time according to the degree of maturation. Dworkin ignores the fact that human fetuses, unlike material artifacts, have the essential potential for interests,[23] and that honoring fetal value may stem from anticipating the interests/rights that will grow out of that potential. We regard early human life, in other words, as a sacred good here and now but also as a future interest-based rights-bearer. Hence social justice is a matter of defending both rights and the necessary conditions for rights. The intrinsic value of fetuses is a necessary (but not a sufficient) condition for interest-based human rights, and we defend that value as a matter of charity and prudence in part precisely to make rights-based justice possible.

Even more importantly, pace Dworkin's step (3), not all rights are based on the interests of extant persons. In the Judeo-Christian tradition in particular, some rights are need based, inhering in both persons and nonpersons. Indeed, it is often the neediness of "nonpersons" that has special claim on us: the lives of the young, the weak, the marginalized, and the diminished take priority as such. We lobby for national health insurance and various social security programs, say, not because they are "deserved" in some meritarian sense, nor even because they are self-consciously wanted, but because they are humanly needed. Moreover, we legislate against child abuse and infanticide not simply because these practices diminish social utility but because they harm vulnerable human beings, beings valuable as such.

If the foregoing is accurate, the killing of a fetus or an incompetent adult may still be unjust even if he or she is not considered a rights-bearer. Again pace Dworkin, it is not the case that justice and injustice are exclusively functions of respect for, or violation of, rights—much less existing personal rights. Justice is a matter of giving individuals their due, but only a narrow liberalism defines what is due exclusively in terms of what others have a present interest-based right to. Would we not call "unjust" a person who secretly used up resources essential to future generations or even who needlessly chopped down a majestic redwood or gratuitously slaughtered the last snail darter? That person would have harmed valuable lives other than his or her own, would have failed to show these lives due reverence, even if we decline to say that he or she has violated any interest-based rights of actual persons. (Though bald eagles are no longer on the endangered species list, we still arrest people who kill them.) Many theists think it unjust to God to destroy a creature willfully (whether in a rain forest or in a human uterus), but atheists as well as theists may think it unjust to the creature itself to take its life, because that life has intrinsic worth or sanctity that ought to be protected . . . and protected legally.

It is by no means a logical or moral necessity even for a liberal democratic society to tie legal protectability entirely to rights and rights entirely to personal interests. Again, many need-based rights and impersonal values are protected in contemporary American law, as in the case of newborns and those with Alzheimer's disease. Think also of future generations and what they are owed; it is often unjust to thwart future persons, and the law properly limits hunting, fishing, and mining rights, for example, to insure that as-yet-unconceived persons are left enough to live on, if not as good as we now have (cf. Locke). If the ability to feel pain is what gives one interests, moreover, rather than the more robust ability to make plans, have hopes, etc., then arguably twelve-week-old fetuses have interests and should be legally protectable. For twelve-week-old fetuses have measurable brain function and the ability to interact discriminately with the uterine environment.[24]

Dworkin would argue that Christians and others are free to make the value judgments they choose in these connections, just not to enforce them legally. As indicated, Dworkin claims that there are two separate questions here: one about inherent value, which is controversial and not to be settled at law in a liberal society, and one about justice and the procedural adjudication of competing interests of persons.[25] This is a false dichotomy, however. Wherever one comes down on abortion, infanticide, intergenerational duties, endangered species legislation, and the like, it is not the case that "grave" questions of the good can be left to individual conscience, while coercion at law can be on "neutral" or purely "reasonable" grounds. To claim that only the interests of extant persons are legally protectable is already to make a controversial value judgment. It may be defensible, but it is not a question of justice free of debatable axiological assumptions, much less a "simple matter of logic," as Dworkin claims. It is not possible to separate judgments of rightness from judgments of goodness; we cannot determine what is just without also determining the goods to be justly produced, preserved, and/or distributed. Indeed, we only understand justice when we have clarified the value of justice itself (e.g., its relation to charity, mercy, even faith). In fact, questions of value precede questions of justice as more basic.

A community's judicial and legislative systems cannot escape acting on some rough social consensus concerning fundamental values and meanings, not excluding the value and meaning of human life. And part of democratic governance involves making room for the volatile educational and conversational processes whereby key axiological issues are publicly debated and acted on. Unanimity will not be had, but there is no escaping the need to hear multiple social voices discussing momentous moral values. Compromise and majority vote, reined in by constitutional checks and balances, will often be the best a democracy can hope for. But the constructive tension that moves a society to ponder the meaning of its shared (and vulnerable) humanity is far preferable to a bogus "pluralism" or "fairness" that claims to prescind from controversial value judgments about life and death. As Gilbert Meilaender has written,

> Especially when we are deliberating the fate of those whom some
> would regard as the weakest and least powerful members of our
> community, whose selfhood might easily be excluded and taken less

seriously, the give and take of political argument is far preferable to the deliberations of a panel that supposes itself to be free of any religious or philosophical perspective.[26]

These words, aimed at President Clinton's Human Embryo Research Panel and its recommendations on abortion and embryo experimentation, are equally relevant to Dworkin et al. and their advice to the Supreme Court on euthanasia and assisted suicide. The fact that most (but not all) candidates for active euthanasia or assisted suicide are competent adults does not negate the reality that they are often weak and vulnerable and that the meaning of their deaths is not a merely "private" affair. Even if a person has reached an assisted death decision in concord with family, friends, and physician, the public effects still go well beyond this circle. When doctors and/or nurses are asked directly and legally to aim at death, via technical means, the meaning of basic caring professions is at stake.

Electoral processes may, after free and open discussion, bring a practice like assisted suicide under legal protection. (This has happened in Oregon but been rejected elsewhere, most recently in Michigan.) But, in that event, the facade of neutrality has been stripped away; those who would dissent have at least had their say and can choose to resist the practice with protests that have been put in religious or philosophical perspective. When, in contrast, appeals to "neutrality" or "tolerance" succeed in foreclosing public debate on a moral issue, civil war may threaten precisely because no real social compromise is possible. In the name of political liberality, the requisite argument and negotiation have been preempted. Substantive opinions cannot be aired as such, so political discussion itself comes to be labeled "fanaticism" or "incivility." In such a context, competing viewpoints can only degenerate into factions that bait and loathe one another, all the while "respecting" one another's "rights." Without a sense of common destiny worked out in open dialogue, we get not the Hobbesian war of all against all but the postmodern peace of none for none.

No doubt, the most telling recent example of political preemption is Harry Blackmun's majority opinion in *Roe v. Wade*. Claiming that "[w]e need not resolve the difficult question of when life begins," Justice Blackmun went on effectively to write fetuses off the rolls of humanity, at least during the first six months of their life.[27] It is not just the substance of the *Roe* decision, let me emphasize, but the manner in which it was or was not justified, that has made elective abortion such an abiding and volatile issue. The point, again, is that to define protectable humanity in terms of the ability to have self-conscious interests is a metaphysically freighted decision—an ethic of "pure dignity"—and once it is made, that decision has profound implications for society as a whole. It is instructive that Peter Singer (like Ronald Dworkin) embraces the interest criterion for personhood, but Singer then judges even one-month-old babies not to have a right to life. Because such babies are not (yet) self-aware, they are effectively the disposable property of their parents. So much for the neutrality and privacy of basic judgments about life and death.

Perhaps the most poignant upshot of their liberal "neutrality" is that Dworkin and his fellow amici are unable legally to protect the necessary conditions for interests and thus for justice itself. There is a strangely self-defeating quality to Dworkin's writings on both elective abortion and assisted suicide, in that he seems to forget that persons only get to be persons and only continue to be persons because they have been extended a care that outstrips strictly adjudicative or meritarian justice. If nascent human beings are to come to have self-conscious interests, and if diminished human beings are to maintain whatever welfare they can, their lives must be valued and protected by society at large. Thus, the survival of justice itself dictates that legal rights cannot be based on extant interests or autonomous choices alone. Needs count, including the need to be valued by others, at both the beginning and the ending of embodied life. So any *amicus curiae* should also, and antecedently, be an *amicus humani generis*.

At the two edges of our existence, sanctity is not a matter of making independent decisions but of receiving and/or giving unearned care, a care that allows us to "go on." All of us begin dependent and in need of suffering love, and all of us (if we live so long) will end dependent and in need of suffering love. There is nothing shameful in this human trajectory; it is the indispensable context of our virtue. The nurturance given infant children by their parents, the attention given the frail and elderly by the young and strong, the forethought given future generations by present persons, etc.—all of these make little or no sense in an ethic of personal dignity alone. We need not sentimentalize human weakness and vulnerability, but we can courageously accept them; we ought not elevate biological animation to the status of summum bonum, but we can refuse to lay violent hands on human life simply because it is not autonomous. (If mere physical life were the highest good, then even passive euthanasia would be wrong.) The point is that liberal justice alone is not enough for a viable, not to mention a good, society. The first virtue, publicly as well as privately, is something very like what Judaism has called "*hesed*," Christianity "*agape*," and Buddhism "the way of compassion." Without embedding justice in a higher virtue like charity, wherein the strong care for the weak, justice itself withers and dies.

In a democratic society many elements of care can be left to generous individuals or philanthropic organizations. Nothing I have written dictates statist solutions to social ills; everything above is compatible with the Catholic doctrine of subsidiarity in which human needs are best addressed by those social bodies (churches, synagogues, clubs, businesses, hospitals) closest to them. Sometimes the coordinating and coercing power of government will be called for, though this power is prudently limited. The fact remains, nonetheless, that basic standing within the moral community and basic furtherance of communal ends cannot be left to "private conscience" or "personal choice" alone, or else the very existence of society is threatened. To repeat, a legal and political commitment to certain shared goods, personal and impersonal, is the necessary condition for justice itself.

Singer endorses the view that infanticide is "the natural and humane solution to the problem posed by sick and deformed babies." He recommends "very strict conditions on permissible infanticide," but these conditions stem almost entirely from concern for the "terrible loss" suffered by adults who happen to "love and cherish the child" and have nothing to do with any inherent wrongness of the act or any intrinsic value of the baby.[28] There is no such wrongness or value, in his opinion. When those closest to a small child do not want it to live, its life is effectively forfeit, since real moral standing requires the capacity for rational desires and self-conscious interests.[29] Neither fetuses nor newborn babies are rational or self-conscious, Singer repeatedly reminds us, so they have no right to life.[30] They are sentient, of course, and Singer admits that conscious pleasures and pains are goods and ills in some sense. But existing personhood trumps so decisively that the only limitation on killing an unwanted, one-month-old child is that it be done without causing suffering—rather like "mercifully" slaughtering a chicken. Singer cannot explain, of course, why parents or anyone else would want to *love* a human babe in arms. The only motivation he has room for here is their stake in their own present emotional gratification or future economic support, but this is not love for the baby him- or herself. It is, rather, an appalling callousness justified in the name of "personhood" and "rationality."

Singer and other hypercognitivists value only present consciousness and self-consciousness; thus they can find no real reason to object to either abortion or infanticide, even when these are done for reasons of parental convenience or social utility.[31] This is tragically forgetful, however, of the temporal trajectory of a human life. One of Singer's central concerns in *Rethinking Life and Death* is to probe the ways in which death may be a process, the phases of which lack clear lines of demarcation. (Higher brain death, permanent loss of the cerebral cortex and limbic system, can come before whole brain death, permanent loss of brain stem function as well. So when do we declare a patient "deceased"?)[32] But he seems oddly oblivious to the ways in which life is a process, requiring different types of care at different times. The oddity is explained when we realize that self-consciousness, here and now, is what matters to Singer, not how we define either death or life. What he is fundamentally "rethinking" is not the definitional criteria for life and death but the moral value and meaning of certain lives and deaths. Even if humans are "living," in some sense, if they lack self-awareness they have little or no significance for Singer—at either end of their historical span, fetal or senile.

Singer's atemporality notwithstanding, it is always salubrious to remember our beginnings in the past care of others (infancy) and to anticipate our likely ends in the future care of others (old age). Such remembrance and anticipation are part of a humility that sees the sanctity in a dependent life, both one's own and another's, and the vanity in a supposedly independent life. For Jews and Christians, the Bible teaches a bracing lesson in this regard: God called creation "good" even before the appearance of sentient beings, including humans (see Gen. 1:4 and 1:12), and God will remain good even after the disappearance of all beings from the face of the earth. Indeed, frequently "what is prized by human beings is an abomination in the sight of God" (Luke 16:15).

Is there any more palpable paradox, any more literal self-contradiction, than Singer's heartfelt concern for persons being coupled with an explicit endorsement of infanticide? Professor Singer now occupies a distinguished chair at Princeton University's Center for Human Values, but the irony of this is unmistakable. His utilitarianism leaves him with little or no sense of the temporal genesis of autonomous personal agents out of dependent impersonal fetuses/babies. He knows human biology, of course, but he is blind to the humane morality that must sustain that biology from beginning to end. There is no question of attributing malice to Peter Singer; he is simply the rock of a new gnostic church that would worship self-awareness and self-control. Even a liberal society must strive for a symbiosis between the goods of dignity and sanctity, however, if it is to address such issues as abortion, infanticide, and euthanasia without self-destructing.

It is hard to say who represents the greater threat to the liberal house, Dworkin or Singer. I recall reading Singer's *Animal Liberation* in the mid-1970s and being impressed with his earnestness and convinced by his moral argument. I am still persuaded by his case against speciesism. He has gone on to take pure dignity to such cruel extremes, however, that he has virtually reductioed his own larger position. However cogent his argument for animal rights, since Singer's utilitarianism implies the moral defensibility of human infanticide and nonvoluntary euthanasia, few liberals have been convinced by it (yet). Many liberals are taken with Dworkin's segregation of "justice/politics" from "value/religion," however, without realizing that it too stems from the valorization of self-consciousness and rational agency. It is tempting, therefore, to see Dworkin as the more subtle eroder of Western principles. Both men are actually gnostics, but Dworkin appears to play the heretic—a friend of liberal democracy who has lost his way and leads others astray with the best of intentions—to Singer's infidel.[33]

The merit of treating Dworkin and Singer together, in any case, is that they highlight each other's "personolatry." If their assumptions are as inadequate as I have argued, both men's visions must be rejected in favor of something rather like agapic love. Whether *agape* requires the theistic convictions of Christian faith is an open question—Buddhism seems the great counterexample—but the primacy of the virtue ought not to be disputed. The reason is simple: the needs and potentials of human lives, which I have associated with sanctity, must be attended to before the choices and achievements of persons, identified with dignity, can be respected.

Conclusion

Familiar Western struggles for social justice have usually centered around efforts to enfranchise a disadvantaged group into the ranks of full personhood. In America, the emancipation of the slaves and the birth of organized labor in the nineteenth century, as well as the securing of civil rights for blacks, women, and gays/lesbians in the twentieth, were movements that focused on the personal dignity of the parties in question. Much remains to be accomplished on these and related fronts, but by demonstrating their subjects' capacity for rational self-governance, these campaigns could militate for their equal membership in the moral community. By and large, even as God helps those who help themselves, democracies have liberated those shown to be already free persons.

Personhood does not spontaneously generate, however, nor, by Christian lights, is individual personhood an end in itself (certainly not the highest). The rational agency associated with autonomous persons is to be used for the sake of ends outside of and larger than the self: most importantly for Christians, love of God and service to the neighbor as fellow creature.[34] The moral keynotes of the last three centuries have been personal liberty and contractual justice precisely because fundamental values like love and creaturely life have been (due to Judaism and Christianity) mostly unquestioned ends. When the liberation of women came to be associated with the right to elective abortion, personal dignity evidently came into conflict with the sanctity of human life. But this is the exception that proves the rule, the transition to something largely new. There is no easy way to balance dignity and sanctity—abortion and euthanasia are real challenges to good conscience—but it is crucial to note the need for some genuine balance.

As we move into the twenty-first century, impersonal values will require a much more explicit articulation and defense. Relations that make possible personal freedom and goods that have a claim on that same freedom are suffering eclipse; the modern ethic of personal dignity has succeeded too well, increasingly leaving us without the wherewithal to recognize and protect human sanctity. Thus is our house divided: not just split, as in Lincoln's day, between two geopolitical camps each claiming legitimacy for its way of life, but tyrannized by a cult of personality that denies virtually all legal standing to what is impersonal. It is vital, and comparatively easy, to warrant that the South's winning the Civil War would have been a calamity for black and other persons; it is less easy, but no less vital, to insist that a similar tragedy is now transpiring for "nonpersons" and thus for all of us who once sojourned as strangers in our mothers' wombs or may yet struggle for memory in hospital wards.[35] When Dworkin et al. maintain in the 1990s that the federal government should be "neutral" on the social status of the very young and the very old, they are mirroring Stephen Douglas's refusal in the 1850s to comment, morally or legally, on the social status of slaves. Douglas wanted to leave the slavery issue to settlement by the individual states, and Dworkin takes this "popular sovereignty" argument one step further in wanting abortion and euthanasia questions to be decided by individuals, period. Lincoln saw that such "liberal" civility is inconsistently applied and finally ethically bankrupt . . . and so should we. (A month-old baby is to Peter Singer what Dred Scott was to Chief Justice Taney: though living for a time in "a free territory," it is still a piece of property to be controlled by its owner[s].)

For all this, a liberalism that would honor human sanctity as well as respect personal dignity is not without resources, even in recent memory. Though difficult to categorize, Simone Weil offers valuable instruction. In a 1943 essay entitled "Human Personality," she writes with the rhetorical elegance and moral authority of a biblical prophet:

> There is something sacred in every man, but it is not his person. Nor yet is it the human personality. It is this man; no more and no less. I see a passer-by in the street. He has long arms, blue eyes, and a mind whose thoughts I do not know, but perhaps they are commonplace. It is neither his person, nor the human personality in him, which is sacred to me. It is he. The whole of him. The arms, the eyes, the thoughts, everything. Not without infinite scruple would I touch anything of this. . . . So far from its being his person, what is sacred in a human being is the impersonal in him. Everything which is impersonal in man is sacred, and nothing else.[36]

The other-regarding implication of this view of sanctity is that we should love and nurture others just as we find them; the self-regarding implication, in turn, Weil takes to be an emphatic ego-negation. "I do not in the least wish that this created world should fade from my view, but that it should no longer be to me personally that it shows itself."[37] Reminiscent of those mystics who favor metaphors of personal extinction over transubstantiation, she makes a virtue of ardent self-effacement. At times she goes too far in this direction and becomes rather masochistic, I fear,[38] but her great merit is to offer a potent remedy for the individualism and rationalism that many associate with Western culture since the eighteenth century. Her own ambivalence about the body makes her acutely sensitive to the fragility of the flesh, as well as of the soul, but she does not despise this. As Weil remarks: "The vulnerability of precious things is beautiful because vulnerability is a mark of existence."[39]

Weil's highlighting of the impersonal dimensions of existence shared by us all can provide clues to a better handling of moral issues ranging from elective abortion to senile dementia. Weilan impersonalism can remind us that fetuses and babies have needs and potentials to be engaged before the dawn of personal consciousness and that Alzheimer patients are capable of a noncognitive well-being to be cared for even after the dusk of rational self-control. Those suffering from end-stage Alzheimer's disease may no longer have either the reality of or the essential potential for autonomous agency, but they manifestly have needs and are still capable of giving and/or receiving love. They have souls, if you will, even if their idiosyncratic selves have withered.[40] As Weil notes, it is the entirety of someone capable of undergoing good and evil, help and harm, that is sacred and commands our attention.[41] And this attention must be social, "rooted" in a moral ethos that acknowledges the situatedness of vulnerable human beings:

> A human being has roots by virtue of his real, active and natural participation in the life of a community which preserves in living shape certain particular treasures of the past and certain particular expectations for the future. This participation is a natural one, in the sense that it is automatically brought about by place, conditions of birth, profession and social surroundings.[42]

A human being's embeddedness in and dependence upon time, chance, and society are not shameful; indeed, human needs and potentials are what make agapic love possible, as well as necessary. That personal autonomy emerges out of impersonal neediness and eventually returns to it is no more scandalous than that an oak tree grows out of an acorn and finally itself falls to the ground. (Falling naturally is not the same as being violently grubbed.) One need only augment Weil's attention to the impersonal with the recognition that we have every reason to preserve both the personal and the impersonal, to treasure both dignity and sanctity. Human sanctity is the seedbed out of which personal dignity flowers, and exalting dignity alone is like wanting to harvest good fruit without cultivating healthy trees. A nation that denies sanctity is divided against itself, to reiterate, uprooted by its own hand.

Notes

1. I have in mind the work of Paul Ramsey, Christopher Lasch, Michael Sandel, Robert Bellah, Steven Tipton, et al. Lasch makes it clear how the "autonomous personality emancipated from custom, prejudice, and patriarchal constraints" has found it hard to see beyond a calculating utilitarianism. See his *The Minimal Self* (New York: Norton, 1984), 205–6.

2. I take the phrase "noncognitive well-being" from Steven G. Post, *The Moral Challenge of Alzheimer Disease* (Baltimore and London: Johns Hopkins University Press, 1995), 9.

3. *New York Review,* March 27, 1997.

4. As I make clear below, this is not to say that all, or even most, deontologists and utilitarians agree on the precise meaning of dignity, but rather that an interesting cross section now focuses on this idea to the neglect of sanctity.

5. I define "active euthanasia" as the direct taking of an innocent human life construed as an act of mercy. This form of euthanasia is to be contrasted with "passive euthanasia," in which an individual is allowed to die by withholding or withdrawing futile or inordinately burdensome treatment. In the active form of euthanasia, the death of the person is intentionally aimed at and either causally brought about or directly facilitated by another; here the party dies because of what is done to her, perhaps by the party herself but with another's help. In the "passive" form of euthanasia, the death is neither willed as an end nor used as a means to some other end, but rather accepted as the upshot of a dying process no longer to be resisted; here the party dies because of an underlying injury or disease, not as the result of self- or other-inflicted assault. As noted below, even when these broad definitions are agreed upon, the moral significance of the acts they describe often is not. One cannot settle the moral debate via terminological fiat, but the above distinctions are important in understanding what is at stake.

6. As long as it remains illegal in most states, the actual incidence of (active) medical euthanasia in the United States will be difficult to determine. The *New York Times* recently reported, however, that "the first national survey to examine how frequently doctors help people kill themselves finds that while patients often ask for help, they rarely get it." "[A] little more than 3 percent" of doctors who care for the seriously ill and dying said that they had written prescriptions for lethal drugs, when asked for by their patients; "and just under 5 percent said they had administered lethal injections to patients on their deathbeds," a figure that includes lethality due to "double effect" as well as direct killing. (See "Assisted Suicides Are Rare, Survey of Doctors Finds," *New York Times,* April 23, 1998, A1.)

7. The *New York Times* quotes a salient observation from Dr. Diane E. Meier, an associate professor of geriatrics at the Mount Sinai School of Medicine and the lead author of the survey referred to in note 6 above: "It is odd that there is such strong public support for legalization of assisted suicide, and we find there is so little of this actually occurring." Also noteworthy is how professional practice and/or conscience might follow law: "When the doctors were asked if they would write lethal prescriptions, defined as assisted suicide, if it were legal, 36 percent said they would. And 24 percent said they would administer lethal injections, defined as euthanasia, if the law permitted it." (See *New York Times,* April 23, 1998, A1.)

8. I say "intelligent free choice" to make clear the self-conscious dimension of dignity; lower animals like fish and fowl are capable of "voluntary" actions, in some sense, but they are not self-aware across time, as far as we know.

9. See, for instance, Glenn Tinder, *The Fabric of Hope: An Essay* (Atlanta, Ga.: Scholars Press, 1999), 179; cf. also Pope John Paul II, *The Splendor of Truth* (*Veritatis Splendor*) (Washington, D.C.: United States Catholic Conference, 1993), 78–84 and 103, and *The Gospel of Life* (*Evangelium Vitae*) (Washington, D.C.: United States Catholic Conference, 1995), passim. In the latter work, the pope frequently refers to the "sacred value" or "sacredness" of human life as well as to "the dignity of the person"—sometimes on the same page (e.g., 5 and 145).

10. Cf. Irving Singer, *The Nature of Love,* vol. 1 (Chicago: University of Chicago Press, 1966).

11. See my *The Priority of Love: Christian Charity and Social Justice* (Princeton: Princeton University Press, 2003), especially chapters 1 and 5.

12. Singer, *Rethinking Life and Death: The Collapse of Our Traditional Ethics* (Oxford: Oxford University Press, 1994), 147.

13. Ibid.

14. See Dworkin, *Life's Dominion: An Argument about Abortion, Euthanasia, and Individual Freedom* (New York: Knopf, 1993), 15–19 and 109–14; and Singer, *Rethinking Life and Death,* 180–83 and 218–19.

15. Dworkin contends that a fetus does not have interests and thus is not a rights-bearer, at least not until very late in pregnancy—roughly thirty weeks of

gestational age. Hence most abortion is not an injustice to the fetus itself, not a violation of its rights. Abortion may be wrong on other grounds, such as the violence it does to the intrinsic value or sanctity of the terminated human life. But the key point is that having intrinsic value does not require or entail having interests, and interests alone are legally protectable in a just society. According to Dworkin, once more, one must not conflate values and interests in arguing about abortion or euthanasia (see *Life's Dominion,* esp. 18). I argue that, on the contrary, the law must attend to both the good and the right, both values and interests, if society is to be either just or loving.

16. See Singer, *Rethinking Life and Death,* e.g., 86 and 93.

17. Ibid., 219.

18. Ibid., 190.

19. Ibid., 130–31.

20. Ibid., 217. Singer has recently had second thoughts about the twenty-eight-day boundary; see his comments in "Dangerous Words," an interview with the *Princeton Alumni Weekly* (January 26, 2000), 19. The problem, however, is not that infanticide is morally wrong in any substantive sense, but rather that the twenty-eight-day cutoff is "too arbitrary" and thus will not "work" as public policy.

21. Singer, *Rethinking Life and Death,* 198; see also 218.

22. Ibid., 208–18.

23. Essential potentials are distinct from mere contingent possibilities. The fulfillment of the former is a matter of growth, the unfolding of intrinsic powers and proclivities, while the realization of the latter requires external manipulation or at least arbitrary luck. Because undamaged human fetuses, with proper care, are disposed to develop self-consciousness, they may be said to have the essential potential for personhood; any given sperm or egg, on the other hand, has only the contingent possibility of contributing to the identity of a person.

24. William P. Smotherman and Scott R. Robinson, "The Uterus as Environment: The Ecology of Fetal Behavior," *Handbook of Behavioral Neurobiology,* vol. 9, ed. E. M. Blass (New York and London: Plenum Press, 1988), 168 and 188.

25. As he puts it, "The crucial question is whether a state can impose the majority's conception of the sacred on everyone" (*Life's Dominion,* 109). His answer is no.

26. Gilbert Meilaender, *Body, Soul, and Bioethics* (Notre Dame: University of Notre Dame Press, 1995), 98–99.

27. See "Roe v. Wade: The 1973 Supreme Court Decision on State Abortion Laws," in *The Ethics of Abortion,* ed. Robert Baird and Stuart Rosenbaum (Buffalo: Prometheus Books, 1989), 18ff.

28. Singer, *Practical Ethics* (Cambridge: Cambridge University Press, 1993), 173.

29. Ibid., 182.

30. Ibid., 183.

31. Ibid., 173–74. For more of Singer's views on these and related topics, see the collection of his essays entitled *Unsanctifying Human Life,* ed. Helga Kuhse (Oxford: Blackwell, 2002).

32. See *Rethinking Life and Death,* especially 20–56.

33. I wish to thank Jon Gunnemann for illuminating discussion of this point, as well as for its phrasing; I do not mean to imply that he agrees with my diagnosis, however.

34. As Robert Kraynak points out, for Thomas Aquinas, for instance, "freedom is only a conditional good that is lawful, right, or licit to the extent that it attains or at least seeks to attain reason's proper end." See Kraynak, "'Made in the Image of God': The Christian View of Human Dignity and Political Order," chapter 3 in this volume. I am more confident than Kraynak about the affinity between Christianity and a (prophetic) form of liberal democracy, but he is surely correct that a Kantian liberalism based on personal autonomy rights is far from the New Testament and the church fathers.

35. On the importance of both remembering and being remembered, morally, see David Keck's *Forgetting Whose We Are: Alzheimer's Disease and the Love of God* (Nashville: Abingdon Press, 1996).

36. Weil, "Human Personality," in *The Simone Weil Reader,* ed. George A. Panichas (Mt. Kisco, N.Y.: Moyer Bell Limited, 1977), 314. I discuss this and related Weilan passages at more length in my *Love Disconsoled: Meditations on Christian Charity* (Cambridge: Cambridge University Press, 1999), 72–79.

37. Weil, *Gravity and Grace,* trans. Emma Craufurd (London and New York: Ark Paperbacks, 1987), 37.

38. See, for example, her so-called "terrible prayer," quoted by Robert Coles in *Simone Weil: A Modern Pilgrimage* (Reading, Mass.: Addison-Wesley, 1987), 131–32.

39. Weil, *Gravity and Grace,* 98.

40. Ted Smith has suggested in conversation that the ability to give or receive loving care—an ability shared by the very young and the very old, the undeveloped and the severely demented—is my better definition of sanctity than one referring to even the potential for autonomy. All human lives have some inherent potential for growth or responsiveness, I believe, but Smith is certainly correct that (1) not all have the potential for rational personhood, as I have defined it, yet (2) they are no less sacred for that. We may love fetuses partially anticipating the selves they will become, even as we may love Alzheimer patients partially remembering the selves they once were. But both sets of human lives are, here and now, souls whose needs have a claim on us.

41. Weil, "Human Personality," 315.

42. See Weil, *The Need for Roots: Prelude to a Declaration of Duties towards Mankind* (London and New York: Ark Paperbacks, 1987), 41.

CHAPTER SIX

Are Freedom and Dignity Enough? A Reflection on Liberal Abbreviations

DAVID WALSH

Political language, Michael Oakeshott has taught us, consists of a set of abbreviations for a far more concretely extended knowledge.[1] This is why politics cannot simply be taught or reduced to a science. It must be picked up in all of its embedded complexity as befits a branch of practical wisdom. Nowhere is this characterization more apt than in the liberal language of rights, which appears to have carried the principle of compression to its limit. "Rights-talk" has become so elliptic that the shorthand is in danger of losing its connection with any sustaining political order. We all know that respect for individual rights is meaningful only in the context of a political order that is capable of preserving them. Yet somehow the core liberal vocabulary of individual rights seems not to invite that wider recognition. As a consequence, liberal politics tends to teeter perpetually on the brink of incoherence and collapse.

The pattern generates an unavoidable anxiety, reflected by a multitude of conferences and anthologies, in which the participants are provoked to wonder if this narrow liberal evocation is capable of surviving. It is a question most eloquently provoked by Glenn Tinder's *Against Fate* in which the underlying tensions are brought to light. Are liberal

abbreviations enough? Or do they necessarily lead to ever shriller demands of a political order that ever fewer are willing to work to preserve? Is the liberal construction an invitation to self-destruction? Or
are there deeper resources within this seemingly fragile arrangement
that might yet rescue us from the threat of disintegration? Are there
depths within the liberal soul of which liberals themselves are scarcely
aware? Such are undoubtedly the questions that press on any observer
of our contemporary political scene in which friction and fracture seem
to shake liberal democracies to their very roots.

Traditionalists have increasingly concluded the situation is hope-
less. The very defenders of the classical liberal ideal, in which individual
liberty is preserved in a constitutional political order, have in many instances lost faith in the project. Not only have liberal democratic polities taken a wrong turn, as conservative voices have argued for half a
century, but that misstep was already implanted in the eighteenth-
century foundation itself. A pluralist political order was a misconcep-
tion in principle. Any construction erected on the principle of removing
conflict from the public to the private realm would inevitably proceed
apace until the public arena had been thoroughly evacuated of all substance. At that point the superstructure could no longer endure and the
house of cards would collapse of its own weight. A critique that began
with a questioning of the legitimacy of public policy has been radi-
calized to cast suspicion on the validity of the entire constitutional
enterprise. Within the United States this means that even the revered
founders are declining in conservative estimation. How, after all, can
they point us toward a deeper wisdom when it is their foundation that
has precisely led toward the dead end of liberal disintegration?[2]

The assessment hardly fares better when we turn to the contemporary standard-bearers of the liberal impulse—the progressive liberals.
They too have moved in the space of fifty years from confidence in the
liberal construction to a state of profound uncertainty concerning its
defensibility. Following the Second World War and its challenge to liberal democratic regimes, a concerted series of attempts to provide a
philosophical articulation of liberal principles culminated in the impressive achievement of John Rawls's *A Theory of Justice* (1971). Within
that work Rawls was able to provide a neo-Kantian justification for the
core principles of liberty and equality within a constitutional order that
respected social differences. His demonstration that "the right is prior

to the good" seemed to have furnished the definitive foundation to the neutral state. But the success was short-lived. Twenty years of critique and reflection were all it took for liberal intellectuals, including Rawls, to concede that the achievement had been overstated. There is no way to articulate a conception of right that utterly avoids taking a position on the good. As a consequence, the project of finding an unassailable defense of rights is exposed as a failure. Incoherence returns to the liberal evocations, and Rawls pleads for an acknowledgement of a politically, if no longer rationally, grounded liberalism. A blunter admission by Richard Rorty insists on the priority of democracy to philosophy and appeals for solidarity despite the manifest contingency of all our liberal convictions. The collapse of liberal faith is transparent.[3]

The burden of the present essay is to suggest that both of these estimations are mistaken. Neither the traditionalist despair nor the postmodern incoherence adequately reflect the enduring and undeniable viability of the liberal political tradition. In the first place both assessments fly in the face of the evident historical durability of such polities. Liberal constitutions have emerged from the competition of modern political forms to outlast and surpass all rivals. Not only did they supersede monarchical and aristocratic forms to establish commercial republics, but they have overcome the far more formidable challenges posed by collectivist and authoritarian rivals in the century just ended. Despite their weakness and unpreparedness liberal democracies found within themselves the resources necessary to defeat fascism and persevere through the long confrontation with communism. Now they stand as the exemplars not only of economic and political success, but as the model of moral legitimacy the world over. No higher aspiration prevails in the contemporary world than to create a political order that is derived from and ordered toward the preservation of individual dignity and respect. The moral and political authority of liberal democratic forms may be ironic, given their own inner self-doubt, but it can hardly be denied as a global reality.

A political form does not demonstrate that kind of world historic persistence without evoking a substantive reality far deeper than the critics' misgivings. Why then the failure to perceive the hidden liberal strength? The reason lies in the misunderstanding of the genre of liberal abbreviations. While it is generally erroneous to take the self-articulation of any political order as a theoretical account of its inner spiritual forces, this is doubly problematic in the case of liberal regimes that have been deliberately fashioned to be as abbreviated as possible. Not only are their principles merely summative of a larger philosophy of existence, but they have been developed to function without explicit reference to that sustaining moral universe. As a consequence liberal political formulations appeal to their self-evidence or, in its absence, seek to function as if the question of foundations did not exist. One of the results of such a strategy is of course that they suggest the non-existence of any broader philosophic or spiritual orientation by which their coherence and conviction are sustained. The superficiality of the pronouncements almost invites the impression that nothing further is entailed. Few observers are prepared to contemplate the possibility that the surface manifestations may conceal a larger underlying reality, from which crises and confrontations can draw forth reserves of virtue surprising even the practitioners themselves. To appreciate this possibility we must examine the structure of liberal political thought.

Minimum Consensus

The first characteristic of a liberal regime is that it is based on a minimal political agreement. Consensus has been narrowed to those principles judged indispensable to the preservation of a common public order. The nature of that judgment may vary over time as elements previously viewed as indispensable are regarded as less momentous. Agreement can continue in the absence of many dimensions previously judged crucial. The most obvious example is of course the early modern struggle over religious or confessional differences. If human beings cannot agree on such fundamental questions as the proper mode of divine worship or of obedience to the divine will, how could agreement be trusted on any lesser matters? Much blood was spilt in the sixteenth and seventeenth centuries in the effort to compel conformity, before the futility of the exercise became apparent. The turning point was formulated in Locke's *Letter on Toleration,* which recognized the inappropriateness of the state attempting to resolve religious differences. Civil society existed for the sake of the political good and could confine itself to the agreement necessary to secure that intermediate end.

The pattern of narrowing the base of consensus had been established. Locke's amplitude of agreement was considerably broader than we would deem necessary, since it excluded atheists and Catholics as unreliable, but it was clearly more limited than what had preceded it. In the centuries that followed other challenges reduced the consensus further, in line with increasing social pluralism. At each stage it has turned out that agreement on the principles of public order can be maintained with a more limited set of background presuppositions. The pattern of increasing social diversification of all types has indeed made the liberal restriction of agreement almost a virtual necessity. It would be difficult to see how a common political order could be maintained in any other way, short of the unlikely possibilities of coercion or persuasion to resolve differences. Far better to focus on those elements of agreement that are indispensable to the maintenance of political society. In our own day the process of consensus shrinkage has perhaps gone so far that many suspect we may have reached the vanishing point. Whether we have is of course the question to be tested here but, before hazarding a conclusion, we should make sure we understand more clearly what is entailed in the conception of a limited consensus.

The impression exists that the principles drawn into such a condensation are unrelated and closed. It is almost as if the bald formulations of rights are taken at face value. Overlooked is the extent to which such declarations represent a selection of the most evocative principles prevailing in the social environment. The liberal invocations of rights, summarizing the necessity of self-determination both individually and collectively, are reflective of the deepest reverence for human dignity. Natural or human rights constitute a recognition of the transcendent worth of each individual, which we are never justified in setting aside in the name of some particular social good. A liberal framework of rights with all of its constitutional prerequisites cannot exist in the absence of that underlying resonance. It is not, therefore, that the liberal principles first exist and then find their connection with some more pervasive understanding of humanity and its place in the order of things. Rather, the liberal invocations emerge with authority only because they are regarded as expressive of the most powerful moral sentiments of a society. They function in this sense, not as self-contained principles of the political order, but as visionary maxims redolent with the deepest and most authoritative intimations of an age.

A deliberately restricted statement of consensus, in the form of mutual guarantees of rights, is therefore not so precarious a foundation as it is often taken to be. On the contrary, it may evince considerable stability as the best expression of the evocative resonances that remain within a context of disagreement and uncertainty. To the extent that the statement of principle represents the authoritative present, it can be the means of arresting further disintegration. A new stage of stability has been reached in which the moving intimations of truth and goodness have found uncontestable expression. Whatever the questions and uncertainties about the broader philosophical framework, this much at least is certain, that human beings deserve to be treated in this way and that political society must be organized on the basis of that recognition. During the sixteenth century it was expressed by Jean Bodin as the realization that friendship between human beings transcended their theological differences; such a recognition of their common humanity was sufficient to provide the substance for a community inclusive of differences.[4] The difficult circumstances culminating in mutual animosity and mistrust once surmounted, in the acknowledgment of mutual humanity, can yield a fairly durable consensus concerning basic obligations despite limited theological explication. Sentiments that had previously sustained a far more elaborate philosophical and theological unfolding now find expression in vaguer but, for that reason, less challenged intellectual expression.

Liberal principles emerge in this way as the residue of resonances that remain of the Christian evocation of the transcendent finality of the person. At the heart of the liberal construction is the recognition of the person as an inexhaustible center of value. When we inquire into the source of this conviction we recognize that it has its most powerful affirmation in the Christian openness of the soul toward God. Through Christ the invitation to participate in the transcendent Being of God is extended to every human being. From this we derive a sense of the uniqueness and unfathomability of every single person. To the extent that each is invited personally to union with God who is the center of all, each human being is already another divine center within the whole order of things. There is no such thing as the good of the whole outweighing the good of the parts when we are dealing with human beings.[5] Each of us is a whole, open to God who is all and in all, and therefore partakers of that transcendent dignity. The liberal language of rights that makes it possible for the good of a single human being to outweigh all social and historical goods is a reflection of that compelling realization. To the extent that the articulation takes place outside of an explicitly Christian context, it represents a secularization of the Christian revelation, but it is not for that reason any the less durable as an acknowledgment of our common self-understanding.

Indeed the very stability of the liberal formulation arises from the residue of Christian resonances that remain within a social setting from which explicit theological reference has largely withdrawn. The rightness of a moral and political language in which the inexhaustible worth of the person is placed at the center still lives from a sense of the movement of participation in the life of God. Discovery of the infinite worth of each human being may take place in this theological framework, but its recognition can endure outside of it. The reason is that Christianity has awakened us to a permanent dimension of human nature which, once differentiated, cannot simply be erased. For anyone with a modicum of spiritual sensitivity the rightness of that perspective remains unarguable. What can be more valuable than a human being? How could we conceive of a social and political good outweighing the rights of a person without undermining the very purpose we seek to serve? If the polity does not reverence the fundamental worth of its members, what else can it serve? These are in a sense Christian sentiments that have migrated to a secular context in which they continue to demonstrate their authoritative truth. Conversely, the secular setting may be viewed as replete with a transcendent orientation on which its very coherence now depends. The lowering of the bar of theological reference entailed by the liberal abbreviated consensus may, but it need not, unfold toward religious indifference or hostility. It may also be a way of preserving spiritual openness with a less substantive theology.

Heightening of Dignity of Person

What makes a secularized spirituality more likely is the second characteristic feature of the liberal construction. Beyond the formation of consensus on implicitly transcendent principles, there is also a distinct heightening of certain aspects of individual dignity. To the extent that all of the weight is placed on the inviolable dignity of the person, there is a corresponding tendency to make that the overarching criterion of moral and political judgment. Autonomy becomes the watchword almost as if its promotion constituted the whole of the moral universe. Anything that obstructs or fetters its unfolding must be removed as anathema to the central conception of what a human being is. It is as free rational beings that we are self-determining and therefore can claim the right to be treated with absolute dignity and respect. No one else can presume to run our lives, not even when they claim to be doing it in our interest. The essence of our humanity requires an umimpeachable recognition of our right to make our own decisions. Anything less would be a catastrophic denial of the dignity of beings that are not only intelligible but also intelligent. It is surely one of the most significant achievements of the liberal philosophical tradition that it has made this recognition a centerpiece of our moral universe of discourse.

By taking the dignity and respect owed autonomous beings as its focus, an important heightening of awareness of its centrality and undeniability has taken place. Liberal moral language marks out the equal dignity and respect owed every human being with dramatic emphasis. A clarity about the criteria for our treatment of one another has been reached through the intensity of focus on the autonomy of the person. It may not provide a fully articulated account of the moral life and clearly stops short of a developed conception of the life of virtue or excellence as the proper fulfillment of a human being. But an unmistakable clarity has been reached concerning the core integrity of the person. Anything that diminishes respect for the inviolability of the person is on its face irreconcilable with the most fundamental conception of what a human being is. Good action is by contrast what enhances the emergence of a community of persons mutually respectful of one another as ends-in-themselves. As Kant formulated it, a rational being must never be regarded as a means but always as determining its own end.[6] This heightened sensitivity to the mistreatment of human beings, which is in many ways the fruit of the liberal concentration on the dignity of the person, has become a significant factor in the movements of social reform that liberal democracies have undertaken in the past two hundred years.

The greater awareness of this central line of emphasis on the person has also been one of the most overlooked sources of its strength. Contrary to the widespread misperception of liberal principles as an inconsequential house of cards, they turn out to have considerable resilience precisely because they are rooted in the sense of constituting a moral advance. While the focus on the person as an inexhaustible center of value is hardly unique to liberal formulations, since it clearly derives from the Christian opening of the soul, the single-minded emphasis imparted to it within the liberal framework has generated its own consequences. Not the least is that it has enabled liberals to mount a critique of the Christian and traditional moralities that had hitherto exercised an authoritative role. In part the success of the liberal analysis is derived from its greater strength as a mode of critique than as a comprehensive account of the moral life; neglect of the more intractable dimensions of human fallenness and the need for reconciliation are nowhere developed. In part too, it must be acknowledged, the liberal critique is convincing within a social environment in which Christian sensitivity to the suffering of the neighbor has often not lived up to its own rigorous demands. But most of all, it is because the liberal identification of the dignity and respect owed every human being constitutes a spotlight of searching intensity. Its power as a moral language derives from its identification of what is in fact the core perspective in which the weighing of private and public actions must be judged. Do they retard or advance the unfolding of our humanity?

The abbreviated character of liberal discourse can be tolerated more readily when it is accompanied by this sense of incontrovertible moral authority. Establishing itself as the primary moral framework occurs, despite its inarticulateness, because it has derived the central illumination from the preceding traditions of philosophy and Christianity. Without the Christian illumination of the transcendent worth of each human being, it would be impossible to conceive the inexhaustible dignity of each individual. Nothing in the world of mundane calculations can explain why human beings alone should escape the logic of instrumentalization.[7] In many ways the exclusivity of the liberal focus on this dignity of self-determination is both its weakness and its strength. Liberal critiques are capable of a searing excoriation of injustice precisely because they deliberately neglect the complexity of context and the ambiguity of motive that continue to define the concrete reality of our lives. The Burkean objection to the abstraction of rights has validity but it overlooks the powerful critical momentum generated by this perspective.[8] Simplification of moral discourse to the essential situation of self-responsibility, while it stands in need of more concrete elaboration, has the inestimable advantage of making the parameters of the human moral situation inescapably clear. Liberal reductions set up an inexorable pressure for reform in line with their elemental sense of right.

Liberal Dependence on Spiritual Traditions

If they are to lead toward substantive enactments and not dissipate their impulse in vacuous idealism, however, the focus on human rights must still draw upon the richer background of spiritual communities and traditions. A militantly secular liberalism can scarcely be sustained. This broader dependence on the differentiated religious traditions, especially Christianity, is the third essential characteristic. While the relationship may be indirect, it is nevertheless crucial. To the extent that the liberal construction represents a secular derivation of the central Christian opening toward transcendent divinity, it is inextricably involved in the relationship with revelation. However, the expression of that relationship can run a wide gamut from the explicitly Christian expression of human dignity to an almost mystical silence before the unfathomability of the person. What is clear is that the transcendent demand for respect cannot be derived from the bald statement of rights. Something more is required as a sustaining force if bills of rights are to be more than "parchment barriers" to the perpetration of injustice. Human proclivities toward the exploitation of others are so persistent that only a correspondingly powerful countermovement can sustain fidelity to the best impulses of our nature. The expression of liberal imperatives may have separated itself from religious language, but their enactment in concrete individual and political existence can hardly dispense with the more robust spiritual traditions. Without the fund of spiritual capital represented by religion, both in its capacity to evoke the summits of self-sacrifice and to surmount the recurrent experiences of human failure and evil, the liberal assertions are prone to shatter under the impact of their own shrillness. The transcendent dignity of the person can only be preserved in its relationship to that which is itself transcendent.

The problem of course is that this dependence is impenetrable from the secular liberal perspective. Convinced of its own rhetoric of independence and endowed with the confidence of its moral superiority, the liberal construction is all too inclined to believe the myth of its own self-sufficiency. As a consequence the relationship of the liberal move- ment to the spiritual tradition whence it received its birth, and on whose sustaining depths it still depends for its resonances, is one of great am- bivalence. On the one hand liberal convictions are imbued with confi- dence in their evocation of the incontrovertible consensus they have reached. The intensity of the focus on autonomous human dignity fur- ther emboldens the liberal mind to contemplate its superiority to all other traditions, including the Christian origins from which it has come. Almost simultaneously, however, liberal reflection becomes aware of its own vulnerability to questions. Without any clear relationship to tran- scendent Being or any developed account of the human trajectory, one has difficulty sustaining the rationale for treating each human being as the only inexhaustible center of value in the universe. In a world defined by instrumental rationality, why should man alone escape the iron ne- cessity of efficiency? The precariousness of the liberal intimations are less an intrinsic feature of the construction than a result of the peculiar myopia within which it tends to operate.

Fragments of Coherence

It is the combination of these three features that together account for the abiding pattern of liberal theory and practice. The liberal political tradition is simultaneously marked by its stability and its instability. The former is evident from its capacity to successfully articulate the bedrock consensus of rightness or fairness in a social context of pluralism and fragmentation. Whatever the issues that divide us, some things remain incontestable. We agree on how we should regard the differences be- tween us because concrete human beings transcend the limits of all their particularities. Beyond the differences we recognize a deeper unity in the common humanity that remains inexhaustible at its core. Whatever the features or attainments of an individual there is always something more to the person, as is the nature of all rational self-governance. The one who does the governing has already gone beyond any stage of self- disclosure and self-enactment he or she has reached. An inescapable dimension of the infinite attaches to each human being and makes each a center of value outweighing the whole world. To the extent that a liberal order of rights gives voice to that ineliminable sense of right, it has attained a bedrock consensus impervious to further movement. But once the insubstantial basis for these convictions is noticed, the sentiment turns quickly to one of greater uncertainty, especially concerning the possibilities for their justification and communication.

Instability then becomes the permanent obverse to liberal stability. It is a pattern that reaches all the way back to the first creators of the liberal abbreviations, most famously John Locke, and bursts forth with renewed anxiety in virtually every generation up to the present.[9] All of the great liberal thinkers from Rousseau to Rawls sensed the vulnerabilities of a set of convictions whose source had deliberately been submerged and which now sought to survive on the basis of their appeal to self-evidence. It was only a matter of time before their justifiability was put in question. How would we respond when someone objected that it was far from self-evident that all men are created equal? Or how would we be able to sustain the conviction that they are endowed with inalienable rights? Would it not make more sense to acknowledge that men and women are, like everything else in reality, inescapably finite? Do they not reach a point where their rights can be alienated once their value to themselves and everyone else has been expended? Why should man be different from every other object under the sun? These are unsettling reflections from a liberal perspective, and the apprehension of their threat has been at the source of the repeated attempts by liberal theorists over the centuries to construct a larger philosophical defense as well as find their way back to some broader religious intuitions. Such a deeper re-evocation of the liberal abbreviations would not only endow it with a more effective intellectual defense but it would also provide it with a means of sustaining the virtues on which its survival depends. Intellectual and moral vulnerabilities unsettle the liberal sense of invincibility and propel its most perceptive advocates into the search for more transparent evocations.

Instability and dissatisfaction with the preceding defenses becomes therefore a permanent feature of the liberal consensus. But anxiety must not be taken as an exclusive or even predominant mood. Equally significant is the equanimity with which the succession of theoretical failures is accepted. The fact that none of the philosophical elaborations has succeeded in establishing its unquestioned primacy is surely indicative of the dimensions of the challenge. But just as impressive is that the theoretical misadventures have not unhinged the underlying certainty of convictions that remain, confident that their rightness has simply not found its most perspicuous elaboration. We may have today reached the limit of such insouciance in the acknowledgment by many such liberal intellectuals that the entire quest for philosophical justification has been an exercise in futility. What is most remarkable about this admission is that it is followed immediately by the recommendation that we carry on with our most cherished convictions without adverting in the slightest to their insubstantiality. "To realize the relative validity of one's convictions and yet stand for them unflinchingly, is what distinguishes a civilized man from a barbarian."[10] Despite the intellectual mendacity of the position, it is difficult to deny the cogency of the contention. To the extent that liberal sentiments have never really lived off a theoretical justification, there is no reason to expect that even the radical collapse of the latter project will overturn the appeal of the former. It is a serious category mistake, Oakeshott has shown, to search among political abbreviations for the source of political convictions. We should rather recognize that the abbreviations are themselves derivative from the practice in which the sentiments that sustain them are activated. This pattern is even more the case with liberal principles that have carried the process of abbreviation virtually to the limits. There would not in fact be the long history of the liberal philosophical quest for transparency if there was not an underlying continuity of sentiments that sustained the search and accepted the limitations of all of the proposed re-evocations. The greatest liberal thinkers, such as Tocqueville or Mill, are marked by the inconclusiveness of their reflections, yet their influence is unaffected by the provisionality of their explications.

What then does the quest for foundations accomplish if it is recurrently frustrated in its goal? Its most enduring achievement is surely that it sustains the awareness of the unencompassable depth of convictions from which the liberal formulations arise. There would be no unending search for foundations if there was not already an awareness of that which provides the foundations. The mere fact of our inability to adequately capture them within the abbreviated language that liberalism imposes on itself does not gainsay the profound presence of such intimations. This is after all the living assurance that supports the indifference to its own theoretical failure. But such failures are never a sheer expense of effort. They are the indispensable paths of reflection by which we approach the inarticulate depths from which the convictions spring. Through the quest for foundations we keep the awareness of foundations alive, and we activate our participation in them most profoundly. Even the embrace of a nonfoundational liberalism, such as we appear to have reached, is not fatal so long as it is not misinterpreted as a sign that foundations are nonexistent. The latter is the mistake of Richard Rorty who counsels us, albeit philosophically, to give up philosophy. Oakeshott, in contrast, represents a more nuanced response that recognizes the failure of philosophical articulation as implying nothing about the presence or absence of animating sentiments. The latter are sufficiently attested both by the continuing practice of liberal politics and by the conviction that guides the search for re-evocation.

Only this recognition of the peculiarly stable instability of the liberal political tradition adequately accounts for the extraordinary profile it exhibits. Its durability and resilience in overcoming the challenges posed against it through a long historical experience have already been noted. What has not been adverted is the extent to which even its most persuasive advocates have often taken the role of friendly critics. It is a tradition or perhaps a non-tradition that seems perpetually in need of being saved from itself. Tocqueville is among the most eminent practitioners of this art as he sifted the American experience to find not only the shape of the future but the means by which it might be saved from itself. "Thus it is," he observed of the extensive associational life of America, "by the enjoyment of a dangerous freedom that the Americans learn the art of rendering the dangers of freedom less formidable."[11] It is no wonder that Tocqueville has become the most admired liberal critic through his harrowing penetration of its flaws, yet he nowhere hints at an alternative or even wistfully sighs for what cannot be. The same is fundamentally true of the twentieth century critics whose standpoint is more firmly rooted in classical and medieval political thought. For all of the enlargement of horizons that has taken place as political theory rediscovered the great fount of wisdom in the past, it has hardly taken on the task of eliminating the liberal public construction. The best for which it can hope is some injection of substance into the incoherence of liberal self-understanding. Even Alasdair MacIntyre, who is presently the most disdainful of liberalism, still retains the hope of reshaping it in line with a more robust Aristotelian tradition.[12]

The stability of the fragmented liberal tradition is perhaps best exemplified by the overarching influence of John Stuart Mill. After Locke he is undoubtedly the figure who most stamps the construction, and it is in his evocation that the shape of liberal self-understanding remains all the way up to the present. Indeed the paucity of major theoretical expositions is striking. With the possible exceptions of Oakeshott and Hayek, there are no intermediate figures of stature between Mill and Rawls. With the latter the re-evocation has become so rarefied philosophically that it has ceased to refer to the full range of political reality and not surprisingly reveals its narrowness in the space of a generation. As a result we still live within the Millian formation of liberal politics. This is most evident in the formulation of the principle of liberty, which strikes us as identifying the appropriate line to justify public interference in the exercise of individual autonomy, i.e., only when it is likely to lead to direct harm to others. But in addition we still struggle with the full range of related issues that Mill adumbrated in his most prominent texts. *On Utilitarianism* is still remarkably close to the principled utilitarian morality around which our public consciousness revolves. *The Principles of Political Economy* proclaims the central struggle between the need for government intervention and the importance of preserving the spirit of private enterprise. We still tinker with the reform of our electoral institutions in order to obviate the problems of mass democracy, as Mill began in *On Representative Government*. Even our confused search for a diffuse humanitarian spirituality is not far away from Mill's late musings on religion. The overarching continuity, however, is that these dimensions of the liberal evocation coexist as unintegrated fragments more or less in the way they coexisted for Mill.[13] Just as they could only be dealt with in separate books, so we too lack any integrating framework through which a comprehensive liberal philosophy might be constructed. The evocative abbreviations continue their quest for a perspicuous framework.

The question that remains for both the defenders and the critics of the liberal configuration is whether the incoherence of its fragments can be relied upon. Are they sufficient to sustain a public order that enhances rather than erodes our fundamental humanity? The question is itself a quintessentially liberal concern. Oscillating between stability and instability the liberal outlook feeds the suspicion that the abbreviations are not enough. Disconnected from their place within a whole the abbreviations are inclined to generate ever more abstract demands that progressively erode the common basis of consensus. Rights-talk becomes the instrument by which an order of rights is cumulatively undermined. Can we therefore place any reliability in a moral and political framework that hardly even seems to be a framework? Does the single-minded focus on autonomy not eventually displace all other conceptions of the good, leading eventually to the evacuation of all substance to the exercise of autonomy itself? If there is nothing worth choosing for its intrinsic goodness, then freedom of choice loses its value.

Such are certainly the tough questions confronting the liberal tradition when the layers of self-assurance are stripped away. But we must not lose sight of the fact that they are posed from within the same tradition, thereby giving evidence of a perspective that goes beyond the preoccupation with autonomy. Such concerns can only have an effect if the preservation of autonomy is already linked with an awareness of a moral order that ultimately measures the use to which liberty is put. However unstated that awareness may be, it is nevertheless there and is ineradicable. To disconnect autonomy from the substantive moral order would be to eliminate its seriousness.[14] Not confined to the routine of instinct, human beings are engaged in the drama of self-disclosure and self-enactment by which they approach what is of transcendent goodness. The abbreviated character of liberal discourse, we now realize, is not truncated speech. Rather, it retains its implicit connectivity to the full range of moral substance drawn into its emphases on autonomy and rights. The whole value of autonomy resonates with its openness to real moral growth. It is a connection that, however it may be obscured or forgotten, cannot be broken without evaporating the very purpose of self-responsibility.

For this reason the priority of the right is less inimical to the order of the good than is often perceived. Far from being mutually opposed, they are inseparable partners. We recall that the dimension of self-responsibility is differentiated in the same context as the recognition of a teleological order of the good. In this sense liberal discourse belies the appearance it may suggest of a part adrift from the larger moral whole; the reality is that it still depends on the context of moral reality whence it has been derived. The major consequence of this recognition is that the unfolding of liberal discourse entails the broader universe of moral discourse. Rights-talk cannot be severed from purpose-talk. We do not, therefore, have to fear disconnection between the two modes of expression, no more than we have to feel that the prominence of autonomy foredooms all other moral considerations. The fragmentary character of rights language still remains, but it is not irretrievably incoherent. Through a patient willingness to explore the confusions, even a certain persistence in pursuing its debates, we will be led to discover the deeper coherence embedded within the framework and which the liberal mind cannot discard without forgoing the source of its own resonance. The liberal language of rights can, in other words, be trusted to disclose and sustain the reality of moral truth.

Coherence Disclosed in Practice

The only condition for the articulation of such a luminous enlargement of rights is that we not lose faith in the encapsulation by the liberal abbreviations of the moral reality of existence. A focus on rights can then become the means of resisting the distortions generated by a misapplication of rights claims. Perhaps the most instructive example of such a reliance on the sufficiency of liberal rights in a moral contest was Lincoln's approach to the institution of slavery. He understood what was widely sensed ever since the Philadelphia Convention, the incompatibility of slavery with the security of rights and self-government. At the same time he was confronted with a long-standing social reality that had acquired legal protection and intellectual justification. Liberal ideology was invoked to protect the rights of property and to insist on the rights of freedom of choice within the states. What is significant about Lincoln's strategy is that he did not despair of the incoherence of the language when confronted with opposing rights claims. He was confident that their irreconcilability could be rendered persuasively. Rather than reverting to some more comprehensive mode of discourse, such as the divine law of the Bible or some variant of natural law, he stuck with the superficially thinner but ultimately evocative terminology of the Declaration of Independence.[15]

The effect was to resuscitate the founding consensus in such a way as to activate its most powerful sentiments. Slavery was confronted with a forthrightness that had been avoided so long as prevailing opinion had hoped it would simply fall away. The necessity had arisen as a result of its expansion, but the mode of confrontation was decisively shaped by Lincoln's leadership. He portrayed it no longer as an unfortunate historical remainder, but as a mortal threat to the very possibility of self-government. Deprivation of the rights of one human being was perceived as an assault on the rights of all. Whatever rags of justification might be invoked under property and choice, the liberty of slave owners, they could not withstand the implication that they undermined the whole possibility of an order of rights. Preservation even of the right of popular liberty cannot be sustained when the choice extends to the derogation of the right of liberty. Slavery is incompatible with the notion of liberty since no one has the right to enslave themselves or others. Freedom is limited by the very presuppositions that make its exercise possible: the presence of self-responsible human beings. Lincoln saw to the depth of the liberal construction, that it is rooted in a moral order from which it cannot detach itself. Even when the abuse of human beings is relatively confined, the damage caused is universal since the abrogation of humanity in one instance eliminates the basis for opposing its extension to all others. Slavery constituted such a radical assault on the basis of liberty that the struggle against it, for all of its destructive consequences, called forth the deepest grounds of the liberal defense. Liberty is most powerfully invoked and illumined when it encounters its greatest threat.

The situation remains the same for us today. Not only has the language of human rights proved a durable and powerful source of the dissident movements that dealt the last blow to the totalitarian incubus, but it continues to be taken up as the sustaining political vocabulary in all contemporary confrontations with tyranny. Even within the established liberal democracies the focus on rights recurrently demonstrates its power of moral conviction. One of the most divisive debates centers around the life issues, especially the legal endorsement of abortion as a right. Undeniably this distortion has a string of mischievous effects as it works its way through the institutions and shapes the codification of rights more broadly. But what is the most effective rhetorical means of opposition? It does not lie in any broadly based moral appeal and especially not on the basis of religious first premises. Such proposals play precisely into the strategy of those who would castigate the prioritization of life as a matter of private or religious disposition and therefore of no relevance in the arena of public argument. No, the most compelling basis for opposing abortion is that of human rights. What is at stake, we may claim, is far more important than any denominational perspective. It is nothing less than the integrity of our public conception of rights. To the extent that the most marginal members of the human species are cast aside, to the same extent does the specter of arbitrariness loom over the notion that any of us are entitled to inviolable dignity and respect. Not only is the language of rights the most publicly persuasive mode of argument; it also evinces the greater moral clarity of its focus on what is owed to human beings simply by virtue of their humanity.

In such demonstrations we begin to discern more clearly the secret of the liberal success as a moral and political form. Fragmentation of principles evokes a minimum consensus, but it also conceals a far deeper integrity of perspective, rooted in the most profound intimation of the transcendent inexhaustiblity of the person. While that unspoken depth cannot be fully articulated, and certainly not through the compressed abbreviations of public exchanges, it can nevertheless be evoked through the intensity of the debates. Liberal formulations may suffer from excessive abbreviation but they do not suffer from a lack of resonance. On the contrary they work as effective symbols of the public order only because their rightness is beyond question. In practice no one stops to request a demonstration of the validity of the proposition that all men are entitled to equal rights. Self-evidence of human rights can provide the public lingua franca only because they guard the full measure of our sense of ourselves and of the mystery in which we exist. Whatever else may be true, of this much at least we can be certain, that we ought to treat one another with ultimate dignity and respect. To doubt the validity of this conviction would be tantamount to undermining the possibility of reflection and discourse. The conviction of rights brings us to the boundary of what can be thought.

Growth of the Soul a Reality

Whence emerges that transcendent imperative within a construction that seems a flat assertion of rights? The answer, and the reason for the impressive resilience of liberal political regimes, is in the practice of the struggle for the right alignment of rights. The liberal practice, we have emphasized, repeatedly calls forth more resources than it seems to possess. The only way in which this is possible is through enacting as a process what is never fully adumbrated in theory. Liberal politics is, as Mark Twain quipped of Wagner's music, better than it sounds. What takes place in the invocation of rights, conscientiously pursued through robust public exchange, is an indefinable growth of the soul that escapes linguistic identification. It is not that further insights are attained or that the social reality is modified in any fundamental way. Growth of the soul is an enlargement of the human beings involved rather than any reality outside of them. All the great liberal thinkers are cognizant of this dimension, and Tocqueville most of all. He refers to the reality repeatedly and isolates "the dangerous exercise of liberty" as the pivotal means for the preservation of liberty. While the change is inner, the effect is far from private. It puts the individual participant in touch with the most real dimension of reality, providing an indubitable sense of contact with what is most enduring. The transformation is that which occurs when ordinarily self-concerned individuals are galvanized into action in the service of what they perceive to be more important than their own private worlds. Suddenly the clarity of purpose and the difficulty of the struggle all become quite secondary. It is not that the inconveniences disappear but they are perceived differently. Now they are measured in the scale of what transcends them because the human beings involved have made contact with a more real reality than what had hitherto dominated their consciousness. Externally nothing is new, but inwardly all is different.[16]

Even the crises that recurrently afflict liberal regimes, many of them self-generated, are thus not the worst outcome. Rightly viewed, the debates that fracture such polities can be the means of promoting a deeper grasp of the principles on which the whole construction depends. A far greater danger is that liberal societies might yield to the temptation to avoid debate. The escapist illusion of a technical or neutral disposition of the differences is always there, even when its appeal has considerably diminished. To eliminate such false escapes altogether it is necessary to see the presence of debate in a far more positive light. What needs to be recognized is that the abbreviations of a liberal order really generate coherent intimations only in the pressure of a struggle with what threatens its core. The presence of robust moral challenges, while they can lead to increasing social cleavages, can also be the means by which they are surmounted in the attainment of a clearer and more firmly held unity. By compelling a liberal order to confront the ambiguities that may have remained unnoticed within it, sharp moral differences can compel the kind of heightening of awareness of the inviolable dignity of the person that lies at the liberal core. The growth of the soul is an event that the incompleteness of a liberal configuration invites and virtually requires as the means of surmounting the tendency toward disintegration. All that is required is the willingness to undertake the struggle and the confidence that below the surface lie unsuspected moral resources for the revitalization of the present. The struggle with its own incoherence is both the necessity and the means by which liberal abbreviations are rendered coherent.

The task of enlarging the liberal soul through engagement with the challenges concretely presented to us does not imply any prediction, pessimistic or optimistic, concerning the outcome. What matters is that the strategy is the only viable one. Not only is the acceptance of the language of rights a pragmatic necessity of public discourse in the present, such acceptance is also morally compelling as well. Despite the abbreviated character of freedom and dignity, they are nevertheless the most appropriate means of confronting the threats of dehumanization that perennially haunt the modern world. Argument on the basis of membership in humanity as such most directly strikes at the attempts to redefine such membership, whether it comes in the form of disregarding the excessively young, infirm, or inconvenient. Once taken up we discover the powerful resonances of all human rights affirmations. Will the appeal be successful? Probably never in any final and definitive way, given the capacity of human beings to find ever new opportunities of dominating others and always under the guise of a new badge of dehumanization. Resistance will always be in the name of defense of the rights of concrete humanity. What is certain is that unless the challenge is taken up, evil will flow unrestricted. Equally certain is that centers of resistance will be forthcoming, since the good too cannot be eliminated from history. The interesting political question is whether such centers of resistance will find an answering response in the wider social reality. Without making any claim to prophecy, I have tried to point toward the unsuspected possibilities of the liberal political tradition rooted in a reverence for the transcendent dignity of the person. At the very least this means that, if liberal polities cannot find their way toward a moral resolution of the conflicts that pervade them, they cannot find their way toward any resolutions at all. Conflict itself remains the most powerful evidence of the moral imperatives that liberal politics cannot discard without also rejecting their own most basic moral commitments.

When seen in the full amplitude of its dynamic the liberal configuration exhibits a very different perspective than that suggested by its customary abbreviations. First, it becomes evident that the respect for individual dignity and autonomy is fully compatible with, although not necessarily cognizant of, the Christian or transcendent worldview. The genius of the liberal arrangement has been to detach itself from all theological reference, but its own performative coherence still strongly depends on the presence of such intimations. The source of such resonance with the inexhaustible depth of the person may remain inarticulate from a liberal perspective, but no one can doubt that this is the dynamic fount of its inspiration. While the lack of explication may be viewed as a dimension of weakness, from another vantage point it is an incalculable strength since it removes the possibility of debilitating critique. That about which we can say nothing, Wittgenstein remarked in one of his wisest comments, we must remain silent. It is that very inarticulateness that guards the mystery of the person from which the liberal dynamic lives.

Second, despite the separation from its Christian background the liberal construction, by virtue of its very narrowness, accomplishes a heightening of the transcendent dignity of the person. There may not be the full amplitude of theological insight concerning man as the *imago Dei* or as the recipient of the redemptive divine outpouring in Christ, but there is a concentration on the inviolability of the individual person. As a consequence the issue of the appropriate treatment of human beings by virtue of nothing more than their humanity becomes a central focus. Without being Christian, it can nevertheless justly claim to have absorbed the Christian valuation of the human being. Concentration on the imperative of respect for human dignity is what imparts to the liberal tradition the sense of constituting a moral advance. This can even extend to the claim of a superior standpoint to Christianity, a claim that depends on a forgetfulness of that which has been heightened. Yet even for the Christian tradition, the differentiation of the liberal focus can provide an invaluable clarification of the direction in which its moral and political influence should be pointed. This is an insight that has not been lost on the Christian churches which now increasingly see the nexus of human rights as the primary focus of their public authority. The inexhaustible dignity and worth of each human being is the point at which the truth of God is most adequately reflected within this world.[17]

The third implication is, therefore, that the liberal order is the closest approximation of the Christian valuation of man. Liberal democracy cannot be regarded as a Christian political form, not only because no political expressions can adequately incarnate the spirit of Christ, but also because it is no longer explicitly connected with its Christian inspiration. A liberal order of rights is more appropriately viewed as a Christian refraction of politics. Like a light penetrating a medium that remains largely unaware of its source, Christianity nevertheless does radiate its illuminative effect. Liberal democracy is a political form that no longer knows the inspiration from which it lives but yet has so condensed its self-understanding that it is able to prevail through its minimum principles. Like much else in our modern world, liberal politics is an expression of anonymous Christianity but is none the less stable for that limited theological exposure. What matters is that the Christian resonances continue to be evoked through a language no longer formally connected with them.

From this recognition follows the fourth implication, that a liberal political order represents in a more profound sense the most adequate political expression of Christianity. The liberal reverence for the dignity of the person is an oblique expression of reverence for that which is the source of human dignity. By naming the transcendent, human language and especially public language already renders it as something immanent. Transcendence cannot be preserved once it is drawn into tangible public expression. Then it suffers the fate of everything finite; it becomes available for manipulation and devaluation. Reverence can be preserved only so long as the inexpressible mystery of God is not reduced to immanent expression. The failure of all political theologies is that they inevitably render the divine as a figure within the partisan conflicts of the day. God is hardly God when he becomes the deity of a particular people or party. He cannot be laid hold of through the clumsy hands of political representation. The best that can be done from a political perspective is to point silently toward that about which our mundane discourse can say nothing. In this way the liberal reverence for the inviolable dignity of the person preserves intact and conveys more powerfully the sense of awe before the mystery by which we are held. There is in this sense a distinct spiritual superiority to liberal reticence.

The only danger is that silence can lapse into ignorance. A fifth implication is that the preservation of the transcendent tension of a liberal order requires a continuing openness to the appropriately transcendent symbolizations of the mystery. Agnosticism and a confused atheism are compatible with a liberal preservation of human dignity, but a dogmatic rejection of the transcendent is not. How can we sustain the notion that each human being is a center of infinite worth if we are certain that there is no such dimension of reality? If the value of every single being can be exhausted then there ceases to be any justification for treating humans as the exception. The rational calculation of costs and benefits must invade everything, consuming even the calculator. An instinctual movement of resistance wells up within us as we contemplate this prospect, but the liberal spotlight on rights strikes us as peculiarly ill-equipped to unfold the rationale for our resistance. For all of the vaunted merits of the liberal essential consensus and the beam of illumination it casts on the indispensability of every human being, it is still not a language in which the development of a meditative self-understanding can take place. Abbreviations may work well in practice but not when the question of theoretical justification arises. Then the liberal compression must look toward what is available in the great spiritual traditions of mankind, those streams in which the deepest and richest effort at self-understanding has taken place. Its own derivation from the resonances of transcendent openness makes liberal reflection a close relative of the world religions, especially Christianity from which it has originated. The viability of liberal convictions depends therefore on the preservation of this relationship of friendship in which it recognizes its own inner filiation. The liberal language of rights may have been developed to avoid the necessity of taking determinate theological positions, but it cannot survive the utter rejection of the value of all theological discourse. Beginning in the conviction that the value of the person matters more than all finite differences, liberal principles still find their deepest confirmation in the movement toward the transcendent God in whom all humanity is united.

Notes

1. Michael Oakeshott, *Rationalism and Politics,* rev. ed. (Indianapolis: Liberty Press, 1991), and also his neglected masterpiece *On Human Conduct* (Oxford: Clarendon Press, 1975).

2. A good recent example of this shift toward a more radical questioning of the liberal democratic tradition was the excitement generated by the *First Things* symposium of November 1996. See *The End of Democracy? The Celebrated* First Things *Debate,* ed. Mitchell Muncy (Dallas: Spence, 1997). The taint of suspicion attaching to the whole liberal tradition is, however, not far from the surface even in such reformist critiques as Mary Ann Glendon, *Rights Talk: The Impoverishment of Political Discourse* (New York: Free Press, 1991), or Michael Sandel, *Democracy's Discontent* (Cambridge: Harvard University Press, 1997).

3. The transition is exemplified by the distance traveled between Rawls's *Theory of Justice* (Cambridge: Harvard University Press, 1971) and his *Political Liberalism* (New York: Columbia University Press, 1993). See also Richard Rorty, *Contingency, Irony and Solidarity* (New York: Cambridge University Press, 1989), and his "The Priority of Democracy to Philosophy," in *The Virginia Statute of Religious Freedom,* ed. Merrill Peterson and Robert C. Vaughan (New York: Cambridge University Press, 1988), 257–82. For an overview, see William Galston, *Liberal Purposes* (New York: Cambridge University Press, 1991).

4. "From this one may learn," he wrote to his friend, Jean Bautru, "that they are mistaken who think agreement on divine matters is necessary in a friendship. For even though Justice, one of the finest virtues, and the good faith between men in society which arises from it, scarcely seem able to exist without religion or dread of some divine powers, nevertheless, the strength and goodness of men's natures are sometimes so great that they are able to draw together in mutual affection men who are unwilling and quarrelsome. . . I had written to you in prior letters to this effect: do not allow conflicting opinions about religion to carry you away; only bear in mind this fact: genuine religion is nothing other than the sincere direction of a cleansed mind toward God." The letter is printed in Paul Lawrence Rose, ed., *Jean Bodin: Selected Writings on Philosophy, Religion and Politics* (Geneva: Droz, 1980), 79–81.

5. One of the most effective brief statements of this principle is contained in Jacques Maritain, *The Person and the Common Good,* trans. John J. Fitzgerald (Notre Dame: University of Notre Dame Press, 1966).

6. Immanuel Kant, *Groundwork of the Metaphysic of Morals,* trans. H. J. Paton (London: Hutchinson, 1948).

7. It is noteworthy that even thinkers who are not particularly sympathetic to religion find themselves compelled to reach back to the language of the sacred

when they wish to convey the unsurpassable dignity that attaches to each human being. Adam Smith, for example, reflecting on the fate of slaves and workers, insists that "the property which each man has in his own labor as it is the original foundation of all other property, so it is the most sacred and inviolable." *The Wealth of Nations,* I.x.c.12.

8. Edmund Burke, *Reflections on the Revolution in France* (Indianapolis: Bobbs-Merrill, 1955) is a powerful critique of the abstraction of the Rights of Man. But it is also a powerful re-evocation of the more substantive historical community that underpins an order of liberty. Interesting parallel critiques of liberal abstractness are provided by Jeremy Bentham and Karl Marx. See the anthology edited by Jeremy Waldron, *Nonsense upon Stilts: Bentham, Burke, and Marx on the Rights of Man* (New York: Methuen, 1987).

9. Locke wrote his famous *Essay Concerning Human Understanding* in large part in response to the difficulty of resolving the moral and religious questions that underlay his conception of civil society. In light of the inconclusiveness of his efforts at philosophic justification he subsequently undertook a reapplication of Christianity that would fulfill the same foundational role in his *On the Reasonableness of Christianity* as well as his later commentaries and paraphrases of the Epistles of St. Paul.

10. This nostrum of Joseph Schumpeter is quoted by Isaiah Berlin in his widely influential essay "Two Concepts of Liberty" as its central thesis. Berlin, *Four Essays on Liberty* (New York: Oxford University Press, 1969), 172.

11. Alexis de Tocqueville, *Democracy in America,* trans. Henry Reeve (New York: Vintage, 1956–58), 2:127.

12. Alasdair MacIntyre, *After Virtue* (Notre Dame: University of Notre Dame Press, 1984).

13. *On Liberty, Utilitarianism, and Considerations on Representative Government* are contained in John Stuart Mill, *On Liberty and Other Essays,* ed. John Gray (New York: Oxford University Press, 1991); *Principles of Political Economy,* ed. Donald Winch (London: Penguin, 1970); *Three Essays on Religion* (Amherst, N.Y.: Prometheus Books, 1998).

14. This is essentially Hegel's critique and development of Kantian morality in *The Philosophy of Right,* trans. T. M. Knox (New York: Oxford University Press, 1967). For a contemporary version of the argument, see Charles Taylor, *The Ethics of Authenticity* (Cambridge: Harvard University Press, 1992) or the more extended account in his *Sources of the Self* (Cambridge: Harvard University Press, 1989).

15. Virtually any of the Lincoln anthologies contain the key selections; see for example *Lincoln on Democracy,* ed. Mario Cuomo and Harold Holzer (New York: Harper, 1991).

16. This insight is the centerpiece of the argument I have explored at greater length in *The Growth of the Liberal Soul* (Columbia: University of Missouri Press, 1997), esp. chapters 6–8.

17. John Paul II has made human dignity the centerpiece of his social teaching and has sought to underpin the language of rights with the more expansive truth of Christ. See especially *Veritatis Splendor* (1993) and *Evangelium Vitae* (1995).

CHAPTER SEVEN

A Well-Ordered Society

JOHN RAWLS

My aim in these remarks is to give a brief account of the conception of equality that underlies the view expressed in *A Theory of Justice* and the principles considered there. I hope to state the fundamental intuitive idea simply and informally; and so I make no attempt to sketch the argument from the original position. In fact, this construction is not mentioned until the end and then only to indicate its role in giving a Kantian interpretation to the conception of equality already presented.

I

When fully articulated, any conception of justice expresses a conception of the person, of the relations between persons, and of the general structure and ends of social cooperation. To accept the principles that represent a conception of justice is at the same time to accept an ideal of the person; and in acting from these principles we realize such an ideal. Let us begin, then, by trying to describe the kind of person we might want to be and the form of society we wish to live in and to shape our interests and character. I shall first describe this notion and then use it to explain a Kantian conception of equality.

First of all, a well-ordered society is effectively regulated by a public conception of justice. That is, it is a society all of whose members accept, and know that the others accept, the same principles (the same conception) of justice. It is also the case that basic social institutions and their arrangements into one scheme (the basic structure) actually satisfy, and are on good grounds believed by everyone to satisfy, these principles. Finally, publicity also implies that the public conception is founded on reasonable beliefs that have been established by generally accepted methods of inquiry; and the same is true of the application of its principles to basic social arrangements. This last aspect of publicity does not mean that everyone holds the same religious, moral, and theoretical beliefs; on the contrary, there are assumed to be sharp and indeed irreconcilable differences on such questions. But at the same time there is a shared understanding that the principles of justice, and their application to the basic structure of society, should be determined by considerations and evidence that are supported by rational procedures commonly recognized.

Secondly, I suppose that the members of a well-ordered society are, and view themselves as, free and equal moral persons. They are moral persons in that, once they have reached the age of reason, each has, and views the others as having, a realized sense of justice; and this sentiment informs their conduct for the most part. That they are equal is expressed by the supposition that they each have, and view themselves as having, a right to equal respect and consideration in determining the principles by which the basic arrangements of their society are to be regulated. Finally, we express their being free by stipulating that they each have, and view themselves as having, fundamental aims and higher-order interests (a conception of their good) in the name of which it is legitimate to make claims on one another in the design of their institutions. At the same time, as free persons they do not think of themselves as inevitably bound to, or as identical with, the pursuit of any particular array of fundamental interests that they may have at any given time; instead, they conceive of themselves as capable of revising and altering these final ends and they give priority to preserving their liberty in this regard.

In addition, I assume that a well-ordered society is stable relative to its conception of justice. This means that social institutions generate an effective supporting sense of justice. Regarding society as a going concern, its members acquire as they grow up an allegiance to the public conception and this allegiance usually overcomes the temptations and strains of social life.

Now we are here concerned with a conception of justice and the idea of equality that belongs to it. Thus, let us suppose that a well-ordered society exists under circumstances of justice. These necessitate some conception of justice and give point to its special role. First, moderate scarcity obtains. This means that although social cooperation is productive and mutually advantageous (one person's or group's gain need not be another's loss), natural resources and the state of technology are such that the fruits of joint efforts fall short of the claims that people make. And second, persons and associations have contrary conceptions of the good that lead them to make conflicting claims on one another; and they also hold opposing religious, philosophical, and moral convictions (on matters the public conception leaves open) as well as different ways of evaluating arguments and evidence in many important cases. Given these circumstances, the members of a well-ordered society are not indifferent as to how the benefits produced by their cooperation are distributed. A set of principles is required to judge between social arrangements that shape this division of advantages. Thus the role of the principles of justice is to assign rights and duties in the basic structure of society and to specify the manner in which institutions are to influence the overall distribution of the returns from social cooperation. The basic structure is the primary subject of justice and that to which the principles of justice in the first instance apply.

It is perhaps useful to observe that the notion of a well-ordered society is an extension of the idea of religious toleration. Consider a pluralistic society, divided along religious, ethnic, or cultural lines in which the various groups have reached a firm understanding on the scheme of principles to regulate their fundamental institutions. While they have deep differences about other things, there is public agreement on this framework of principles and citizens are attached to it. A well-ordered society has not attained social harmony in all things, if indeed that would be desirable; but it has achieved a large measure of justice and established a basis for civic friendship, which makes people's secure association together possible.

II

The notion of a well-ordered society assumes that the basic structure, the fundamental social institutions and their arrangement into one scheme, is the primary subject of justice. What is the reason for this assumption? First of all, any discussion of social justice must take the nature of the basic structure into account. Suppose we begin with the initially attractive idea that the social process should be allowed to develop over time as free agreements fairly arrived at and fully honored require. Straightaway we need an account of when agreements are free and the conditions under which they are reached are fair. In addition, while these conditions may be satisfied at an earlier time, the accumulated results of agreements in conjunction with social and historical contingencies are likely to change institutions and opportunities so that the conditions for free and fair agreements no longer hold. The basic structure specifies the background conditions against which the actions of individuals, groups, and associations take place. Unless this structure is regulated and corrected so as to be just over time, the social process with its procedures and outcomes is no longer just, however free and fair particular transactions may look to us when viewed by themselves. We recognize this principle when we say that the distribution resulting from voluntary market transactions will not in general be fair unless the antecedent distribution of income and wealth and the structure of the market is fair. Thus we seem forced to start with an account of a just basic structure. It's as if the most important agreement is that which establishes the principles to govern this structure. Moreover, these principles must be acknowledged ahead of time, as it were. To agree to them now, when everyone knows their present situation, would enable some to take unfair advantage of the social and natural contingencies, and of the results of historical accidents and accumulations.

Other considerations also support taking the basic structure as the primary subject of justice. It has always been recognized that the social system shapes the desires and aspirations of its members; it determines in large part the kind of persons they want to be as well as the kind of persons they are. Thus an economic system is not only an institutional device for satisfying existing wants and desires but a way of fashioning wants and desires in the future. By what principles are we to regulate a scheme of institutions that has such fundamental consequences for our view of ourselves and for our interests and aims? This question becomes all the more crucial when we consider that the basic structure contains social and economic inequalities. I assume that these are necessary, or highly advantageous, for various reasons: they are required to maintain and to run social arrangements, or to serve as incentives; or perhaps they are a way to put resources in the hands of those who can make the best social use of them; and so on. In any case, given these inequalities, individuals' life-prospects are bound to be importantly affected by their family and class origins, by their natural endowments and the chance contingencies of their (particular early) development, and by other accidents over the course of their lives. The social structure, therefore, limits people's ambitions and hopes in different ways, for they will with reason view themselves in part according to their place in it and take into account the means and opportunities they can realistically expect.

The justice of the basic structure is, then, of predominant importance. The first problem of justice is to determine the principles to regulate inequalities and to adjust the profound and long-lasting effects of the social, natural, and historical contingencies, particularly since these contingencies combined with inequalities generate tendencies that, when left to themselves, are sharply at odds with the freedom and equality appropriate for a well-ordered society. In view of the special role of the basic structure, we cannot assume that the principles suitable to it are natural applications, or even extensions, of the familiar principles governing the actions of individuals and associations in everyday life which take place within its framework. Most likely we shall have to loosen ourselves from our ordinary perspective and take a more comprehensive viewpoint.

III

I shall now state and explain two principles of justice, and then discuss the appropriateness of these principles for a well-ordered society. They read as follows:

1. Each person has an equal right to the most extensive scheme of equal basic liberties compatible with a similar scheme of liberties for all.
2. Social and economic inequalities are to meet two conditions: they must be (a) to the greatest expected benefit of the least advantaged and (b) attached to offices and positions open to all under conditions of fair opportunity.

The first of these principles is to take priority over the second, and the measure of benefit to the least advantaged is specified in terms of an index of social primary goods. These goods I define roughly as rights, liberties, and opportunities, income and wealth, and the social bases of self-respect. Individuals are assumed to want these goods whatever else they want, or whatever their final ends. The least advantaged are defined very roughly, as the overlap between those who are least favored by each of the three main kinds of contingencies. Thus this group includes persons whose family and class origins are more disadvantaged than others, whose natural endowments have permitted them to fare less well, and whose fortune and luck have been relatively less favorable, all within the normal range (as noted below) with the relevant measures based on social primary goods. Various refinements are no doubt necessary, but this definition of the least advantaged suitably expresses the link with the problem of contingency and should suffice for our purposes here.

I also suppose that everyone has physical needs and psychological capacities within the normal range, so that the problems of special health care and of how to treat the mentally defective do not arise. Besides prematurely introducing difficult questions that may take us beyond the theory of justice, the consideration of these hard cases can distract our moral perception by leading us to think of people distant from us whose fate arouses pity and anxiety. Whereas the first problem of justice concerns the relations among those who in the normal course of things are full and active participants in society and directly or indirectly associated together over the whole course of their life.

Now the members of a well-ordered society are free and equal; so let us first consider the fittingness of the two principles to their freedom, and then to their equality. These principles reflect two aspects of their freedom, namely, liberty and responsibility, which I take up in turn. In regard to liberty, recall that people in well-ordered society view themselves as having fundamental aims and interests which they must protect, if this is possible. It is partly in the name of these interests that they have a right to equal consideration and respect in the design of their society. A familiar historical example is the religious interest; the interest in the integrity of the person, freedom from psychological oppression and from physical assault and dismemberment is another. The notion of a well-ordered society leaves open what particular expression these interests take; only their general form is specified. But individuals do have interests of the requisite kind and the basic liberties necessary for their protection are guaranteed by the first principle.

It is essential to observe that these liberties are given by a list of liberties; important among these are freedom of thought and liberty of conscience, freedom of the person, and political liberty. These liberties have a central range of application within which they can be limited and compromised only when they conflict with other basic liberties. Since they may be limited when they clash with one another, none of these liberties is absolute; but however they are adjusted to form one system, this system is to be the same for all. It is difficult, perhaps impossible, to give a complete definition of these liberties independently from the particular circumstances, social, economic, and technological, of a given well-ordered society. Yet the hypothesis is that the general form of such a list could be devised with sufficient exactness to sustain this conception of justice. Of course, liberties not on the list, for example, the right to own certain kinds of property (e.g., means of production), and freedom of contract as understood by the doctrine of laissez-faire, are not basic; and so they are not protected by the priority of the first principle.[1]

One reason, then, for holding the two principles suitable for a well-ordered society is that they assure the protection of the fundamental interests that members of such a society are presumed to have. Further reasons for this conclusion can be given by describing in more detail the notion of a free person. Thus we may suppose that such persons regard themselves as having a highest-order interest in how all their other interests, including even their fundamental ones, are shaped and regulated by social institutions. As I noted earlier, they do not think of themselves as unavoidably tied to any particular array of fundamental interests; instead they view themselves as capable of revising and changing these final ends. They wish, therefore, to give priority to their liberty to do this, and so their original allegiance and continued devotion to their ends are to be formed and affirmed under conditions that are free. Or, expressed another way, members of a well-ordered society are viewed as responsible for their fundamental interests and ends. While as members of particular associations some may decide in practice to yield much of this responsibility to others, the basic structure cannot be arranged so as to prevent people from developing their capacity to be responsible or to obstruct their exercise of it once they attain it. Social

arrangements must respect their autonomy and this points to the appropriateness of the two principles.

IV

These last remarks about responsibility may be elaborated further in
connection with the role of social primary goods. As already stated,
these are things that people in a well-ordered society may be presumed
to want, whatever their final ends. And the two principles assess the
basic structure in terms of certain of these goods: rights, liberties, and
opportunities, income and wealth, and the social bases of self-respect.
The latter are features of the basic structure that may reasonably be
expected to affect people's self-respect and self-esteem (they are not the
same) in important ways.[2] Part (a) of the second principle (the difference principle, or as economists prefer to say, the maximin criterion)
uses an index of these goods to determine the least advantaged. Now
certainly there are difficulties in working out a satisfactory index, but I
shall leave these aside. Two points are particularly relevant here: first,
social primary goods are certain objective characteristics of social institutions and of the people's situation with respect to them; and second,
the same index of these goods is used to compare everyone's social circumstances. It is clear, then, that although the index provides a basis for
interpersonal comparisons for the purposes of justice, it is not a measure of individuals' overall satisfaction or dissatisfaction. Of course, the
precise weights adopted in such an index cannot be laid down ahead
of time, for these should be adjusted, to some degree at least, in view of
social conditions. What can be settled initially is certain constraints on
these weights, as illustrated by the priority of the first principle.

Now, that the responsibility of free persons is implicit in the use
of primary goods can be seen in the following way. We are assuming
that people are able to control and to revise their wants and desires in
the light of circumstances and that they are to have responsibility for
doing so, provided that the principles of justice are fulfilled, as they are
in a well-ordered society. Persons do not take their wants and desires as
determined by happenings beyond their control. We are not, so to speak,
assailed by them, as we are perhaps by disease and illness so that wants
and desires fail to support claims to the means of satisfaction in the way
that disease and illness support claims to medicine and treatment.

Of course, it is not suggested that people must modify their desires and ends whatever their circumstances. The doctrine of primary goods does not demand the stoic virtues. Society for its part bears the responsibility for upholding the principles of justice and secures for everyone a fair share of primary goods (as determined by the difference principle) within a framework of equal liberty and fair equality of opportunity. It is within the limits of this division of responsibility that individuals and associations are expected to form and moderate their aims and wants. Thus among the members of a well-ordered society there is an understanding that as citizens they will press claims for only certain kinds of things, as allowed for by the principles of justice. Passionate convictions and zealous aspirations do not, as such, give anyone a claim upon social resources or the design of social institutions. For the purposes of justice, the appropriate basis of interpersonal comparisons is the index of primary goods and not strength of feeling or intensity of desire. The theory of primary goods is an extension of the notion of needs, which are distinct from aspirations and desires. One might say, then, that as citizens the members of a well-ordered society collectively take responsibility for dealing justly with one another founded on a public and objective measure of (extended) needs, while as individuals and members of associations they take responsibility for their preferences and devotions.

V

I now take up the appropriateness of the two principles in view of the equality of the members of a well-ordered society. The principles of equal liberty and fair opportunity (part (b) of the second principle) are a natural expression of this equality; and I assume, therefore, that such a society is one in which some form of democracy exists. Thus our question is: by what principle can members of a democratic society permit the tendencies of the basic structure to be deeply affected by social chance, and natural and historical contingencies?

Now since we are regarding citizens as free and equal moral persons (the priority of the first principle of equal liberty gives institutional expression to this), the obvious starting point is to suppose that all other social primary goods, and in particular income and wealth, should be equal: everyone should have an equal share. But society must take organizational requirements and economic efficiency into account. So it is unreasonable to stop at equal division. The basic structure should allow inequalities so long as these improve everyone's situation, including that of the least advantaged, provided these inequalities are consistent with equal liberty and fair opportunity. Because we start from equal shares, those who benefit least have, so to speak, a veto; and thus we arrive at the difference principle. Taking equality as the basis of comparison those who have gained more must do so on terms that are justifiable to those who have gained the least.

In explaining this principle, several matters should be kept in mind. First of all, it applies in the first instance to the main public principles and policies that regulate social and economic inequalities. It is used to adjust the system of entitlement and rewards, and the standards and precepts that this system employs. Thus the difference principle holds, for example, for income and property taxation, for fiscal and economic policy; it does not apply to particular transactions or distributions, nor, in general, to small scale and local decisions, but rather to the background against which these take place. No observable pattern is required of actual distributions, nor even any measure of the degree of equality (such as the Gini coefficient) that might be computed from these.[3] What is enjoined is that the inequalities make a functional contribution to those least favored. Finally, the aim is not to eliminate the various contingencies, for some such contingencies seem inevitable. Thus even if an equal distribution of natural assets seemed more in keeping with the equality of free persons, the question of redistributing these assets (were this conceivable) does not arise, since it is incompatible with the integrity of the person. Nor need we make any specific assumptions about how great these variations are; we only suppose that, as realized in later life, they are influenced by all three kinds of contingencies. The question, then, is by what criterion a democratic society is to organize cooperation and arrange the system of entitlements that encourages and rewards productive efforts? We have a right to our natural abilities and a right to whatever we become entitled to by taking part in a fair social process. The problem is to characterize this process.[4]

At first sight, it may appear that the difference principle is arbitrarily biased towards the least favored. But suppose, for simplicity, that there are only two groups, one significantly more fortunate than the other. Society could maximize the expectations of either group but not both, since we can maximize with respect to only one aim at a time. It seems plain that society should not do the best it can for those initially more advantaged; so if we reject the difference principle, we must prefer maximizing some weighted mean of the two expectations. But how should this weighted mean be specified? Should society proceed as if we had an equal chance of being in either group (in proportion to their size) and determine the mean that maximizes this purely hypothetical expectation? Now it is true that we sometimes agree to draw lots but normally only to things that cannot be appropriately divided or else cannot be enjoyed or suffered in common.[5] And we are willing to use the lottery principle even in matters of lasting importance if there is no other way out. (Consider the example of conscription.) But to appeal to it in regulating the basic structure itself would be extraordinary. There is no necessity for society as an enduring system to invoke the lottery principle in this case; nor is there any reason for free and equal persons to allow their relations over the whole course of their life to be significantly affected by contingencies to the greater advantage of those already favored by these accidents. No one had an antecedent claim to be benefited in this way; and so to maximize a weighted mean is, so to speak, to favor the more fortunate twice over. Society can, however, adopt the difference principle to arrange inequalities so that social and natural contingencies are efficiently used to the benefit of all, taking equal division as a benchmark. So while natural assets cannot be divided evenly, or directly enjoyed or suffered in common, the results of their productive efforts can be allocated in ways consistent with an initial equality. Those favored by social and natural contingencies regard themselves as already compensated, as it were, by advantages to which no one (including themselves) had a prior claim. Thus they think the difference principle appropriate for regulating the system of entitlements and inequalities.

VI

The conception of equality contained in the principles of justice I have described is Kantian. I shall conclude by mentioning very briefly the reasons for this description. Of course, I do not mean that this conception is literally Kant's conception, but rather that it is one of no doubt several conceptions sufficiently similar to essential parts of his

doctrine to make the adjective appropriate. Much depends on what one
counts as essential. Kant's view is marked by a number of dualisms, in
particular, the dualisms between the necessary and the contingent,
form and content, reason and desire, and noumena and phenomena. To
abandon these dualisms as he meant them is, for many, to abandon what
is distinctive in his theory. I believe otherwise. His moral conception
has a characteristic structure that is more clearly discernible when these
dualisms are not taken in the sense he gave them but reinterpreted and
their moral force reformulated within the scope of an empirical theory.
One of the aims of *A Theory of Justice* was to indicate how this might
be done.

   To suggest the main idea, think of the notion of a well-ordered
society as an interpretation of the idea of a kingdom of ends thought of
as a human society under circumstances of justice. Now the members
of such a society are free and equal and so our problem is to find a rendering of freedom and equality that is natural to describe as Kantian;
and since Kant distinguished between positive and negative freedom,
we must make room for this contrast. At this point I resorted to the
idea of the original position: I supposed that the conception of justice
suitable for a well-ordered society is the one that would be agreed to
in a hypothetical situation that is fair between individuals conceived
as free and equal moral persons, that is, as members of such a society.
Fairness of the circumstances under which agreement is reached trans-
fers to the fairness of the principles agreed to. The original position
was designed so that the conception of justice that resulted would be
appropriate.

   Particularly important among the features of the original position
for the interpretation of negative freedom are the limits on information,
which I called the veil of ignorance. Now there is a stronger and a
weaker form of these limits. The weaker supposes that we begin with
full information, or else that which we possess in everyday life, and then
proceed to eliminate only the information that would lead to partiality
and bias. The stronger form has a Kantian explanation: we start from
no information at all; for by negative freedom Kant means being able
to act independently from the determination of alien causes; to act from
natural necessity is to subject oneself to the heteronomy of nature. We
interpret this as requiring that the conception of justice that regulates
the basic structure, with its deep and long-lasting effects on our com-

mon life, should not be adopted on grounds that rest on a knowledge
of the various contingencies. Thus when this conception is agreed to,
knowledge of our social position, our peculiar desires and interests, or
of the various outcomes and configurations of natural and historical
accident is excluded. One allows only that information required for a
rational agreement. This means that, so far as possible, only the general
laws of nature are known together with such particular facts as are
implied by the circumstances of justice.

Of course, we must endow the parties with some motivation, otherwise no acknowledgment would be forthcoming. Kant's discussion in
the *Groundwork* of the second pair of examples indicates, I believe, that
in applying the procedure of the categorical imperative he tacitly relied
upon some account of primary goods. In any case, if the two principles
would be adopted in the original position with its limits on information, the conception of equality they contain would be Kantian in the
sense that by acting from this conception the members of a well-ordered
society would express their negative freedom. They would have succeeded in regulating the basic structure and its profound consequences
on their persons and mutual relationships by principles the grounds for
which are suitably independent from chance and contingency.

In order to provide an interpretation of positive freedom, two
things are necessary: first, that the parties are conceived as free and equal
moral persons must play a decisive part in their adoption of the conception of justice; and second, the principles of this conception must
have a content appropriate to express this determining view of persons
and must apply to the controlling institutional subject. Now if correct,
the argument from the original position seems to meet these conditions.
The assumption that the parties are free and equal moral persons does
have an essential role in this argument; and as regards content and
application, these principles express, on their public face as it were, the
conception of the person that is realized in a well-ordered society. They
give priority to the basic liberties, regard individuals as free and responsible masters of their aims and desires, and all are to share equally in the
means for the attainment of ends unless the situation of everyone can
be improved, taking equal division as the starting point. A society that
realized these principles would attain positive freedom, for these principles reflect the features of persons that determined their selection and
so express a conception they give to themselves.

Notes

Reprinted by permission of the author, John Rawls. Originally published in *The Cambridge Review* (February 1975), pp. 94–99, as "A Kantian Conception of Equality." Reprinted as "The Well-Ordered Society" in *Philosophy, Politics, and Society,* ed. Peter Laslett and James Fishkin (New Haven: Yale University Press, 1979).

1. This paragraph confirms H. L. A. Hart's interpretation. See his discussion of liberty and its priority, *Chicago Law Review,* April 1973, pp. 536–40.

2. I discuss certain problems in interpreting the account of primary goods in "Fairness to Goodness," *Philosophical Review,* October 1975, pp. 536–54.

3. For a discussion of such measures, see A. K. Sen, *On Economic Inequality* (Oxford, 1973), chap. 2.

4. The last part of this paragraph alludes to some objections raised by Robert Nozick in his *Anarchy, State, and Utopia* (New York, 1974), esp. pp. 213–29.

5. At this point I adapt some remarks of Hobbes. See *The Leviathan,* chap. 15, under the thirteenth and fourteenth laws of nature.

CHAPTER EIGHT

Saving Modernity from Itself: John Paul II on Human Dignity, "the Whole Truth about Man," and the Modern Quest for Freedom

KENNETH L. GRASSO

Contrary to what is occasionally suggested, the ideas of freedom and human dignity are not discoveries of the modern world. In fact, as has been pointed out countless times, these ideas figure prominently in the biblical vision of the person and are a constitutive element of Christian anthropology. It is nevertheless true, however, that with the rise of modernity, they come to assume a new importance, a new prominence. Walter Kasper expresses a commonplace when he observes that in the modern era "mankind in its freedom and its worth becomes the point of departure, and the middle and end point of thought."[1]

In the social and political arenas, this exaltation of the freedom and dignity of the person has created widespread ferment by prompting a far-reaching desire for the transformation of social life so as to make it conform more fully to man's dignity. Politically, this ferment has given birth to a new type of polity. The hallmarks of what might be called the free society are its commitments to the idea of human rights, to religious, intellectual, artistic and scientific freedom, to equality before the law, and to the right of the people to participation in public affairs. These commitments, in turn, find expression in the idea of constitutional democracy, of government that is limited in its scope, subject in its operations to the rule of law, and responsible to those it governs.

John Paul's understanding of the dignity of the human person emerges out of his engagement with the modern quest for human dignity and freedom. The key to grasping his posture toward this quest is the recognition that, in Charles Taylor's terminology, John Paul is neither one of modernity's "knockers" nor one of its "boosters."[2] Rejecting both the type of uncompromising antimodernism toward which Catholic thought often tended prior to the Second Vatican Council and the type of uncritical embrace of modern culture which has been so influential among Western Catholic intellectuals in the decades since the Council, John Paul, as Kenneth L. Schmitz notes, "calls upon the Church neither wholly to endorse nor wholly to condemn modernity."[3]

A proper evaluation of modernity, John Paul insists, must reckon with modernity in its full complexity, and thus take cognizance of both the ways in which the modern world embodies affirmations and values rooted in the Christian vision of man and reality, and the ways in which it departs from the vision. In its confrontation with modernity, therefore, the Catholic mind must recognize and assimilate both the legitimate aspirations and accomplishments of the modern world and "the fundamental achievements of modern and contemporary thought,"[4] while seeking to purify them of whatever in them is incompatible with Christian truth.

Thus, John Paul by no means simply rejects the modern turn to the subject or exaltation of human freedom and dignity. "Modern philosophy," he affirms, "clearly has the great merit of focusing attention upon man"(FR, 5, 13), and has "enriched" our "heritage of knowledge and wisdom in different fields" (FR, 91, 112). Likewise, he applauds the fact that there is no "social or political programme in today's world in which man is not invariably brought to the fore," no "social, economic, political or cultural programme" that would fail to describe itself as "humanistic."[5] Indeed, he praises the contemporary world's "great desire for political, social and economic institutions which will help individuals and nations to affirm and develop their dignity."[6]

Indeed, as even the most cursory survey of his writings will reveal, John Paul's thought is animated by a passionate concern for the freedom and dignity of the human person. In fact, in a letter to his friend, the eminent Jesuit theologian Henri de Lubac, written shortly after he became a cardinal in 1968, he remarked that "I devote my very rare free moments to a work that is close to my heart and devoted to the metaphysical sense and mystery of the person."[7] It is no accident that John Paul's thought has been described by one of its leading interpreters as a "Christian humanism."[8]

If John Paul applauds the modern celebration of the dignity and freedom of the human person, this is not to suggest that he believes modernity has achieved its goal of making "every element of this life correspond to man's true dignity" (RM, 14, 45), of establishing a type of society "worthy of the person."[9] On the contrary, he fears that certain deep-seated currents in modern life and thought threaten this freedom and dignity. Indeed, "the evil of the times," he wrote de Lubac, "consists in the first place in a kind of degradation, indeed in a pulverization, of the fundamental uniqueness of each human person. This evil is even much more of the metaphysical order than of the moral order."[10]

Ironically, as his reference to "the metaphysical order" suggests, John Paul believes that if human freedom and dignity are today threatened, this is to a significant degree due to the way in which this freedom and dignity have been understood by modern thought. At the heart of the problems that beset the modern world, he contends, is a flawed conception of the nature and foundations of man's dignity and freedom, the effect of which has been to deform and frustrate the modern world's quest for a social order "worthy of the human person."[11]

Confronted with the crisis that threatens it today, John Paul does not call for the abandonment of the modern quest for freedom but rather seeks to rescue it from modernity's own self-subverting and ultimately self-destructive tendencies. This, he argues, will require correcting and purifying the very metaphysics of the person that has informed modern thought and thus will involve nothing less than the "'recapitulation' of the inviolable mystery of the person."[12]

I

On innumerable occasions in the course of his papacy, John Paul has invoked the opening sentences of a text he has hailed as one of the

foundational documents of contemporary Catholic social teaching: the
Second Vatican Council's Declaration of Religious Freedom. "A sense
of the dignity of the human person," the Declaration begins,

> has been impressing itself more and more deeply on the con-
> sciousness of contemporary man. And the demand is increasingly
> made that men should act on their own judgment, enjoying and
> making use of a responsible freedom, not driven by coercion but
> motivated by a sense of duty. The demand is also made that con-
> stitutional limits should be set to the powers of government, in
> order that there may be no encroachment on the rightful freedom
> of the person and of associations. This demand for freedom in
> human society chiefly regards the quest for the values proper to the
> human spirit. It regards, in the first place, the free exercise of reli-
> gion in society.[13]

Commenting approvingly on the developments referred to in this
passage, John Paul affirms that "the *full awareness* among large numbers
of men and women of their own dignity and of that of every human
being" represents one of the "*positive* aspects" of our times.[14] Indeed,
"this heightened sense of the dignity of the human person and of his or
her uniqueness, and of the respect due to the journey of conscience, certainly represents one of the positive achievements of modern culture."[15]

It should be emphasized here that this appeal to human dignity is
no mere rhetorical gambit. The idea of man's dignity as a person lies
at the heart of John Paul's vision, emerging as one of the central themes
of both John Paul's philosophical personalism and the Christocentric
anthropology that inform his thought. On the one hand, the recognition that human beings are persons brings with it a recognition of their
dignity, their natural greatness, the recognition that they hold "a position superior to the whole of nature" and stand "above everything else
in the visible world."[16] On the other hand, "in Christ and through
Christ," as he proclaims in his first encyclical, *The Redeemer of Man*,
"man has acquired full awareness of his own dignity, of the heights to
which he is raised, of the surpassing worth of his own humanity"
(RM, 11, 32). The "almost divine dignity" of the human person,[17] he has
tirelessly insisted, is an integral part of the Gospel message and hence

of the Church's teaching (RM, 12, 36). Indeed, the dignity of the human is nothing less than "the basic good of collective and individual life" (PC, 180).

Nor is John Paul hesitant about embracing the implications of modern man's heightened sense of the dignity of the human person. "One of the distinguishing marks of our times," he notes, is a "universal longing for freedom."[18] Far from lamenting this longing, John Paul celebrates it, echoing the Second Vatican Council's affirmation that the people of our day are right to value freedom highly and "pursue it eagerly."[19] The "quest for freedom," in fact, arises inexorably "from a recognition of the inestimable dignity and value of the human person," and the consequent desire "to be given a place in social, political and economic life . . . commensurate with" this dignity.[20]

The connection between the recognition of man's dignity as a person and the quest for freedom is not mysterious. Here again, John Paul echoes the Council's Pastoral Constitution on the Church in the Modern World. "Authentic freedom," the Council affirms, is "an exceptional sign of the divine image in man."[21] "By giving man an intelligent and free nature," John Paul notes,

> God has thereby ordained that each man alone will decide for himself the ends of his activity, and not be a blind tool of someone else's ends. Therefore, if God intends to direct man towards certain goals, he allows him . . . to know those goals, so that he may make them his own and strive toward them independently. In this amongst other things resides the most profound logic of revelation: God allows man to learn his supernatural ends, but the decision to strive towards an end, the choice of course, is left to man's free will. God does not redeem man against his will.[22]

In the Council's formulation, "God has willed that man be left 'in the hand of his own counsel' . . . so that he can seek his creator spontaneously, and come freely to utter and blissful perfection through loyalty to Him."[23] Man's dignity therefore requires him to seek truth and goodness through a choice that is "personally motivated and prompted from within," not under "blind internal impulse," or "mere external pressure."[24] Inasmuch as inherent in man's dignity as a person is an exigence to act on his or her own responsibility and initiative, this dignity demands that the freedom of the human person be respected. To respect the dignity of the human person, therefore, it is necessary to respect human freedom.

This dignity, in turn, is the source of an order of "'human rights'—rights inherent in every person and prior to any Constitution and state legislation" (EV, 18, 34), "rights . . . inscribed by the Creator in the order of creation."[25] The human person, John Paul proclaims, by virtue of his "transcendent dignity . . . as the visible image of the invisible God, is . . . by his very nature the subject of rights which no one may violate—no individual group, class, nation or State. Not even the majority of a social body may violate these rights. . . ."[26] Our fundamental rights therefore are inalienable because they are grounded not on social convention but on our intrinsic dignity. As such, "they precede all social conventions and provide the norms that determine their validity."[27] The growing recognition of man's dignity as a person, therefore, finds expression "in the . . . lively concern that human rights should be respected, and in the . . . vigorous rejection of their violation."[28]

Thus, the long historical process that led to the discovery of this idea must be hailed as one of the greatest achievements of the modern age (EV, 18, 34). Celebrating the United Nations' Universal Declaration of Human Rights as "one of the highest expressions of the human conscience of our time,"[29] John Paul insists that "the common good . . . is brought to full realization only" when "the objective and inviolable rights of man" are respected (RM, 17, 63). Indeed, he affirms that "to the Gospel message belong all the problems of human rights."[30]

At the institutional level, John Paul's solicitude for the freedom and rights of the human person translates into an embrace of the institutions and practices of constitutional democracy. "The free and responsible participation of all citizens in public affairs," "the rule of law," and "respect for and promotion of human rights" are essential to "the 'health' of a community." Thus, wherever conditions allow, the well-being of the body politic requires the establishment of "democratic and participatory" forms of government.[31] In fact, "democracy" is to be numbered among "the most precious and essential goods of society" (EV, 70, 115). Thus, "if today we see an almost universal consensus with regard to the value of democracy, this is to be considered a positive 'sign of the times,' as the Church's Magisterium has frequently noted" (EV, 70, 115). Indeed, during a trip to Latin America early in his papacy he observed that "if democracy means human rights"—if it means a political system rooted in and dedicated to the rights of the person—"it also belongs to the message of the Church."[32]

II

It should be obvious that John Paul exhibits a genuine admiration for the principles, institutions, and practices that together compose the modern ideal of the free society. (Any remaining doubts on this score can be dispelled by examining his comments regarding the foundations of the American democratic experiment.)[33] At the same time, however, he is at pains to call attention to the shadows that today fall upon the free societies of the modern West. Not limited to the specific moral shortcomings of these societies, his concerns extend to the public philosophy—the understanding of the intellectual and moral foundations of the free society—that has come to inform their public life. On the one hand, he laments that "nowadays there is a tendency to claim that agnosticism and skeptical relativism are the philosophy and the basic attitude which correspond to democratic forms of political life."[34] Relativism, it is held, is "an essential condition of democracy, inasmuch as it alone" can "guarantee tolerance, mutual respect between people and acceptance of the decisions of the majority." The idea of objective and binding moral truth, in contrast, leads inexorably to "authoritarianism and intolerance" (EV, 70, 114).

Alongside this emerging "alliance between democracy and relativism" (VS, 101, 123), we have witnessed the growth of "a completely individualistic conception of freedom," a conception of freedom "which exalts the isolated individual in an absolute way" (EV, 19, 36). Government, in this view, exists to protect the moral autonomy of individuals, to safeguard their right to be subject to no moral norms not of their own making. Respect for this autonomy, in turn, demands that government "should not adopt or impose any ethical position but [instead must] limit itself to guaranteeing maximum space for the freedom of each individual, with the sole limitation of not infringing on the freedom . . . of any other citizen" (EV, 69, 113).

These trends, John Paul is convinced, represent a grave threat to the future of the free society and the authentic values it embodies. Indeed, the threat they pose is so grave that he wonders at one point if we have not arrived at a turning point in the long historical process that culminated in the establishment of these societies (EV, 18, 34).

"The value of democracy," he maintains, "stands or falls with the values which it embodies and promotes." Democratic institutions are "a means and not an end." Their value derives from their capacity to embody and promote certain goods, fundamental among which are "the dignity of every human person, respect for inviolable and inalienable human rights, and the adoption of the 'common good' as the end and criterion regulating political life." "The basis of these values," furthermore, "cannot be provisional and changeable 'majority' opinions, but only the acknowledgment of an objective moral law" (EV, 70, 115).

Democracy, therefore, "is only truly such when it acknowledges and safeguards the dignity of every human person" (EV, 20, 38). The development of a sound democracy thus requires the affirmation of "those essential and innate human and moral values which flow from the very truth of the human being and express and safeguard the dignity of the person: values which no individual, no majority and no state can ever create, modify or destroy, but must only acknowledge, respect and promote" (EV, 71, 116). It is these values which find expression in the demands of the objective and universal moral law. And because these values constitute nothing less than the moral foundation of democratic government, the acknowledgement of the "universal and unchanging" demands of the moral order represents "the unshakeable and solid guarantee of a just and peaceful human coexistence, and hence of genuine democracy" (VS, 96, 118).

By denying the existence of such an order, relativism simultaneously reduces our intrinsic dignity and fundamental rights to the status of mere "social conventions" and deprives us of an "objective standard to help adjudicate different conceptions of the personal and common good."[35] By depriving politics of an objective moral grounding (EV 70, 116), relativism strikes at the very foundations of democratic government. Without a "sure principle for guaranteeing just relations between people,"[36] democracy is "reduced to a mere mechanism for regulating different and opposing interests on a purely empirical basis" (EV 70, 115) and "democratic politics to a raw contest for power."[37] Under such conditions, law becomes nothing more than an expression of "the will of the stronger part" (EV, 20, 38), and "force . . . becomes the criterion for choice and action in . . . social life" (EV, 19, 36). Under such conditions, "democracy . . . becomes an empty word" because "the democratic ideal . . . is betrayed in its very foundations" (EV, 70, 116).

Thus, far from serving the cause of the dignity and rights of the person, when conceived in a relativistic fashion, democracy "easily turns into open or thinly disguised totalitarianism."[38] In fact, moral relativism prevents a society from answering "questions [that are] fundamental to a democratic political community," such as "Why should I regard my fellow citizen as my equal? Why should I defend someone else's rights? Why should I work for the common good?" Insofar as "democracy cannot be sustained without a shared commitment to certain moral truths about the human person and human community," John Paul concludes, a climate of moral relativism ultimately makes democracy impossible.[39]

Similar dangers accompany the radically individualistic conception of freedom that has emerged in recent decades. Insofar as it makes "freedom . . . absolute in an individualistic way," this conception ignores human freedom's "essential link to the truth" and "inherently relational dimension." By "giving no place to solidarity, to openness to others and service to them," it leads to a rejection of our responsibilities toward others (EV, 19, 36–37). It thereby issues in

> a serious distortion of life in society. If the promotion of the self is understood in terms of absolute autonomy, people inevitably reach the point of rejecting one another. Everyone else is considered an enemy from whom one has to defend oneself. Thus society becomes a mass of individuals placed side by side, but without any mutual bonds. Each one wishes to assert himself independently of the other and in fact intends to make his own interests prevail. Still, in the face of other people's analogous interests, some kind of compromise must be found, if one wants a society in which the maximum possible freedom is guaranteed to each individual. In this way, any reference to common values and to a truth absolutely binding on everyone is lost, and social life ventures on to the shifting sands of complete relativism. At that point, everything is negotiable, everything is open to bargaining. (EV, 20, 37–38)

In practice, therefore, this "completely individualistic concept of freedom ... ends up becoming the freedom of 'the strong' against the weak"
(EV, 19, 36–37). Thus, although superficially attractive, this view "ultimately destroys the personal good of individuals and the common good
of society." "Freedom as autonomy," John Paul writes,

> by its single-minded focus on the autonomous will of the individual
> as the sole organizing principle of public life, dissolves the bonds of
> obligation between men and women, parents and children, the strong
> and the weak, majorities and minorities. The result is the breakdown
> of civil society, and a public life in which the only actors of conse-
> quence are the autonomous individual and the state. This, as the 20th
> century ought to have taught us, is a sure prescription for tyranny.[40]

III

The obvious question here concerns how these tragic developments can
be explained. Although John Paul praises modernity's heightened sensitivity to the dignity and freedom of the person, he simultaneously
laments that "this perception, authentic as it is, has been expressed in
a number of more or less adequate ways, some of which however di-
verge from the truth about man as a creature in the image of God, and
thus need to be corrected and purified in the light of faith" (VS, 31,
47–48). The crisis that assails the modern ideal of the free society is
rooted in the very conception of human dignity and freedom that has
historically undergirded it, and ultimately in the very metaphysics of
the person that lies at the heart of modern thought.

The deepest root of the confusion that plagues modern man is
found in "the eclipse of the sense of God" characteristic of "a social and
cultural climate dominated by secularism" (EV, 21, 39). "Only by admit-
ting his innate dependence," his status as "a creature to whom God has
granted being and life as a gift and a duty," is it possible for man to "live
and use his freedom to the full, and at the same time respect the life and
freedom of every other person" (EV, 96, 151).

"When the sense of God is lost," however, "there is also a tendency
to lose the sense of man," to lose sight of "the mystery" of man's own
being (EV, 22, 42). "When God is forgotten," writes John Paul echo-

ing the Constitution on the Church in the Modern World, "the creature itself grows unintelligible" (EV, 22, 40). The loss of God issues in
a profound misunderstanding of the nature of the human person, which
finds expression in practical materialism, individualism, utilitarianism,
and hedonism (EV, 23, 42). Thus, "when God is denied and people live
as though he did not exist, . . . the dignity of the human person" also
ends "up being rejected or compromised" (EV, 96, 151). "The eclipse of
the sense of God" thus constitutes "the heart of the tragedy being
experienced by contemporary man" (EV, 21, 39).

If the loss of the sense of God and of man is the ultimate cause of
the crisis besetting the free societies of the modern West, the immediate cause is the far-reaching "crisis of truth" (VS, 32, 48) that assails
contemporary thought. While "modern philosophy clearly has the great
merit of focusing attention upon man," this very focus tends to create
a one-sided emphasis on human subjectivity. The result is "an ever-
deepening introversion," which acts to lock "the human spirit . . . within
the confines of its own immanence without reference of any kind to the
transcendent" (FR, 5, 13–14) and culminates in the denial that the human
mind is "equipped to know the truth and to seek the absolute" (FR, 47,
64). The ultimate result of this crisis of truth is a "nihilism" that is at
once "the denial of all foundations and the negation of all objective
truth" and that ultimately leads "either to a destructive will to power
or to a solitude without hope" (FR, 90, 111).

This crisis has profound implications. Its rejection of objective truth
strikes at the very ground of human dignity (FR, 90, 111) and reduces
the orders of justice and human rights to the status of mere social conventions. Under its impact, moreover, we have witnessed the emergence
of a new conception of freedom. Untethered from truth, freedom is
exalted "almost to the point of idolatry" (VS, 54, 73) and elevated to
the status of an "absolute" (VS, 32, 48). It thus comes to enjoy "a primacy
over truth, to the point that truth itself" comes to be considered a "creation of freedom" (VS 35, 51). This absolutization of freedom thus fos-
ters an individualistic ethos wherein each individual possesses "his or
her own truth, different from the truth of others" (VS, 35, 51). In fact,
taken to its extreme consequences, this individualism leads to a denial
of the very idea of human nature (VS, 32, 49).

Absolutized in this fashion, "freedom alone, uprooted from all
objectivity" (VS, 84, 106) becomes the source of values (VS, 32, 48),

laying "claim to a moral autonomy" which "would actually amount to an absolute sovereignty" (VS, 35, 51–52). As a result, the individual conscience is granted "the prerogative of independently determining the criteria of good and evil" (VS, 32, 48). At the moral level, therefore, this radically individualistic ethos finds expression in the rejection of "the idea of the universal truth about the good, knowable by human reason" (VS, 32, 48), of the "idea that there exists a moral law inscribed in our humanity, which we can come to know by reflecting on our nature and our actions, and which lays certain obligations upon us because we recognize them as universally true and binding." Indeed, the very idea of such a law is a violation of the rights of conscience, an abrogation of freedom.[41]

Thus, at the center of the crisis of moral culture[42] that today threatens the free society is the detachment of freedom from "its essential and constitutive relationship to truth" (VS 4, 13)." When freedom, out of a desire to emancipate itself from all forms of tradition and authority," writes John Paul,

> shuts out even the most obvious evidence of an objective and universal truth, which is the foundation of personal and social life, then the person ends up by no longer taking as the sole and indisputable point of reference for his own choices the truth about the good and evil, but only his own subjective and changeable opinion or, indeed, his selfish interest and whim. (EV, 19, 37)

Such a conception of freedom effectively absolutizes the will of the individual or the group by granting to the one or the other *"the right to determine what is good and evil"* (VS, 35, 51).

It thereby reduces politics to nothing more than a struggle for power, thereby effectively legitimizing the oppression and exploitation of the weak by the strong. Thus, "when freedom is detached from objective truth it becomes impossible to establish personal rights on a firm rational basis; and the ground is laid for society to be at the mercy of the unrestrained will of individuals or the oppressive totalitarianism of public authority" (EV, 16, 151). Indeed, totalitarianism arises precisely from a "denial of truth in the objective sense" and the consequent "rejection of an objective criterion of good and evil beyond the will of those in power."[43] When its essential link to the truth is severed, in short, "freedom negates and destroys itself, and becomes a factor leading to the destruction of others" (EV, 19, 37).

Freedom, therefore "is not simply the absence of tyranny or oppression." Nor is it "license to do whatever we like." On the contrary, freedom has a "moral structure," an "inner architecture," which must be respected if it is to exist. Freedom, this is to say, possesses

> an inner "logic" which distinguishes it and ennobles it: freedom is ordered to the truth, and is fulfilled in man's quest for truth and in man's living in the truth. Detached from the truth about the human person, freedom deteriorates into license in the lives of individuals, and, in political life, it becomes the caprice of the most powerful and the arrogance of power.[44]

As the grim events of the twentieth century confirm, "once the truth is denied to human beings, it is pure illusion to try to set them free. Truth and freedom go together hand in hand or together . . . perish in misery" (FR, 90, 111).

IV

The fatality that has plagued the modern quest for freedom flows from within modernity itself. It stems from the flawed metaphysics of the person through which modernity has conceptualized this dignity and its demands and the tragic misunderstanding of the moral structure of freedom[45] in which this metaphysics issued. It is this flawed metaphysics that has distorted and frustrated the modern world's quest for freedom. Inasmuch as true freedom is possible "only . . . on the basis of a correct conception of the human person and of the person's unique value,"[46] the task confronting modernity is the purification and correction of its quest for freedom in the light of "the whole truth about man" (RM, 12, 36).

Inasmuch as a comprehensive account of this truth would involve a systematic survey of John Paul's thought, only its very broadest outlines may be sketched here.[47] To begin with, "since it is metaphysics which makes it possible to ground the person's dignity" (FR, 83, 104), an adequate understanding of the human person and his or her dignity necessarily involves an adequate metaphysics of the person. The starting point and essential foundation of such a metaphysics of the person must be "the philosophy of being" as that philosophy has been understood within the Christian metaphysical tradition (FR, 97, 119). By virtue of its metaphysical and moral realism, this philosophy provides a secure foundation for humanity's "capacity to *know the truth,* to come to knowledge which can reach objective truth by means of that *adequatio rei et intellectus*" (FR, 82, 113). At the same time, "based upon the very act of being itself," the philosophy of being "allows a full and comprehensive openness to reality as a whole, surpassing every limit in order to reach the one who brings all things to fulfillment" (FR, 97, 120). By virtue of its "genuinely metaphysical" orientation (FR, 83, 104), it is uniquely equipped to address the ultimate and overarching meaning of life (FR, 81, 102).

To suggest that an adequate metaphysics of the person must begin from and operate in the overarching framework of the philosophy of being is not to imply that it limit itself to sterile repetition of the formulas of a particular thinker or tradition of thought. On the contrary, the philosophy of being must assimilate the insights of the entire philosophical tradition (FR, 97, 119). In particular, to forge an adequate metaphysics of the person, the philosophy of being must assimilate "the fundamental achievements of modern and contemporary thought" (FR, 84, 107).

It is true, of course, that modern philosophy "has taken wrong turns and fallen into error" (FR, 49, 66). Indeed, its embrace of an exaggerated rationalism (FR, 41, 65) has brought it into conflict with Christian revelation and produced the crisis of truth and meaning we witness. At the same time, however, "a good part of modern and contemporary philosophy would not exist without the stimulus" of Christian revelation. This stimulus includes "the Christian proclamation of human dignity, equality and freedom," which "has undoubtedly influenced modern philosophical thought" (FR, 76, 96–97). And, whatever errors may vitiate it, it is undeniable that modern philosophy has enriched our wisdom and knowledge through its "analyses of perception and experience, of the imaginary and the unconscious, of personhood and intersubjectivity, of freedom and values, of time and history" (FR, 64, 112).

Thus, an adequate metaphysics of the person must assimilate into the philosophy of being "the precious and seminal insights" (FR, 48, 64) of contemporary and modern philosophical thought. In John Paul's view, the most important of these insights center on the whole question "of the subjectivity of the human being" (PC, 209). The traditional Aristotelian anthropology, which shaped important aspects of the philosophy of being's approach to human nature, defined man as a rational animal. "This definition," he notes, "fulfills Aristotle's requirements for defining the species (human being) through its proximate genus (living being) and the feature that distinguishes the given species in that genus (endowed by reason)" (PC, 210).

Although the usefulness of this definition is unquestionable, it brings with it certain risks. Embodying an understanding of man as "one of the objects in the world to which the human being visibly and physically belongs," it implies—at least at first glance—a belief in the reducibility of the human being to the world. The problem is that "the human being's proper essence cannot be totally reduced to and explained by the proximate genus specific difference" (PC, 211).

What such a "cosmological" understanding of the person fails to do justice to is "the human being's complete uniqueness in the world" (PC, 210). It fails to do so because it ignores the human being's status "as a concrete self, a self-experiencing subject," a being which experiences "its acts and inner happenings, and with them its own subjectivity" (PC, 213). "It is not enough," he maintains, "to define a man as an individual member of the species" because "there is something more to him, a particular richness and perfection in the manner of his being" which "cannot be wholly contained within the concept 'individual member of the species'" (LR, 22). A human being is not simply an individual specimen of the human species—a human being is "a personal subject," "a unique and unrepeatable" self (PC, 214).

This dimension of man's nature can only be approached "inwardly." It can only be disclosed or revealed through the "lived experience," and hence the consciousness, of the human person (PC, 215). Inasmuch as this "lived experience essentially defies reduction," it is necessarily overlooked by the type of metaphysical interpretation or reduction (PC, 213) characteristic of the cosmological approach with its "species definition of man" and its "belief that the essentially human is basically reducible to the world," that the human being can be adequately understood mainly as an object, as one of the objects existing in the natural world (PC, 211). "The primordial uniqueness of the being" (PC, 211)—"the great gulf which separates the world of persons from the world of things" (LR, 21), from the other entities which comprise the natural world—cannot be adequately grasped by an approach that limits itself to understanding man "as an objective being" (PC, 210). On the contrary, man's proper essence can only be grasped by an approach that recognizes *"the basic irreducibility of the person to the natural world"* and thus understands man's nature in light of his subjectivity, his lived experience of self-possession and self-governance (PC, 211, 214).

If John Paul denies that what he terms the cosmological approach can provide us with a fully adequate understanding of human nature, this is not to suggest that he believes it is completely mistaken. On the contrary, it provides us with access to important truths about human nature and plays an indispensable role in securing the metaphysical foundations for the selfhood of the human person. Indeed, without it, the truths conveyed by the cosmological approach, the understanding of man as a person, would appear doomed to veer toward a thoroughgoing subjectivism and ultimately toward an annihilation of the subject (PC, 220).

Given the important truths it conveys, it follows that just as we cannot arrive at an adequate conception of the human being via the cosmological approach alone, so also we cannot do so while remaining within the framework of the irreducible subject alone. We cannot arrive at an adequate understanding of human nature while remaining within the horizon of the human person's experience of his or her subjectivity alone for the simple reason that while remaining within this horizon we are "unable to get beyond the pure self" (PC, 214); we remain trapped in the subjective consciousness of the person.

The key to grasping John Paul's metaphysics of the person is the recognition that he believes that far from being irreconcilable the two approaches are ultimately complementary. Thus, the disclosure of the personal subjectivity of the human being "need in no way signify a break with reduction and the species definition of the human being" for the simple reason that "the personalistic type of understanding of the human being is not the antinomy of the cosmological type but its complement" (PC, 213). Inasmuch as each brings to light a distinctive dimension of human existence, a true and complete picture of the human being must draw on both the cosmological and the personalistic approaches to the understanding of human nature. In an adequate

anthropology, each of these approaches "must be cognitively supple-
mented with the other" (PC, 214).

Thus, as John F. Crosby points out, John Paul does not seek to
replace the cosmological understanding of man characteristic of the
Aristotelian tradition, which analyzes "human beings . . . in terms of
substance, potentiality, rationality, and the like." Rather, he seeks to
complete it both by exploring dimensions of human existence that the
latter tradition gives short shrift to and showing how the truths contained in the cosmological approach "are in fact understood more deeply
through the personalist approach," which gives special attention to personal subjectivity and analyzes man in categories such as "interiority,
self-presence, self-donation."[48] John Paul's metaphysics of the person
has as its goal the "enrichment of the realistic image of the person" (PC,
220) through the assimilation into the framework of the philosophy of
being of the legitimate insights regarding the subjectivity of the person
contained in modern philosophies of freedom and consciousness.

It is against the backdrop of this metaphysics of the person that
John Paul's conception of human dignity takes shape. In the created
world, he affirms, the human person is the most perfect being, *perfec-
tissimum ens* (PC, 167). To begin with, this dignity is a function of man's
nature as a person, his nature as "an individual being of a rational nature
(*individua substantia rationalis naturae*)," to employ Boethius's famous
definition (LR, 22). As a person, man, in the words of the Declaration
on Religious Liberty, is "endowed with reason and free will and therefore privileged to bear responsibility."[49] These characteristics, in turn,
attest to man's nature as a spiritual being, to the spiritual character of
the human soul (PC, 168). Thus, if by virtue of our bodies we are a mere
speck in the vast created universe, the fact is that by virtue of our souls
we transcend the whole material world.[50]

Man's nature thus differs fundamentally from that of not only in-
animate objects and plants, but from that of animals as well. Only man
is capable of conceptual thinking (LR, 22). Only a human being can
think and speak and through "language express the beauty of art and
poetry and music and literature and the theater."[51] Only a human being
can grapple with the problems of truth and goodness, can inquire into
the ultimate cause of everything, and how to "possess goodness at its
fullest" (LR, 23).

Likewise, man differs from all these others by virtue of the fact that he alone acts from choice, that he alone possesses "the power of self-determination." This means that each person must decide for himself the ends of his activity (LR, 24, 27). We must freely choose through our actions to strive for the perfection of humanity through the performance of morally good actions (VS, 39, 55). Man's personhood thus implies a task and involves a grave responsibility. Indeed, John Paul invokes Saint Gregory of Nyssa, noting insofar as by our actions we shape our very selves, "*we are* in a certain way our own parents, creating ourselves as we will, by our decisions" (VS, 71, 91). Human actions thus not only manifest the self, but also constitute the person, and thus possess an "autoteleological" character (PC, 230).

In the final analysis, however, man's dignity cannot be adequately appreciated as long as one approaches man cosmologically. Although it is a unique and unrepeatable entity, it nevertheless suffices to view an individual animal simply as a single specimen of a particular species. A man, however, cannot be wholly contained within the concept "individual member of the species." He cannot be contained within this horizon because "there is something more to him, a particular richness and perfection in the manner of being" (LR, 21–22). Each human being, this is to say, "has the particular 'specific gravity' of a personal being"—of a personal self, in each instance unique and unrepeatable" (PC, 237). Thus, if when "an individual perishes, the species remains unaltered," the fact is that "when a person dies, something unique and unrepeatable is lost."[52] Only when seen against this backdrop can the singular dignity of each and every human being be understood.

A full appreciation of the dignity, the greatness, of the human person, however, only becomes possible in the light of divine revelation. Revelation, as the Constitution on the Church in the Modern World affirms, opens up vistas closed to human reason.[53] At the same time, it both confirms truths readily accessible to human reason and "proposes certain truths which might never have been discovered by reason unaided, although they are not of themselves inaccessible to reason" (FR, 76, 96). To begin with, the dignity of the human person finds confirmation in the very fact of divine revelation, in the very fact that God speaks to man, that God establishes contact between himself and man and communicates to man his own thoughts and plans (PC, 179). This call, moreover, is addressed not to some men or to humanity in general, but to each and every person.

This dignity implicit in the fact of revelation receives further confirmation in revelation's content. Through revelation, we discover man's unique relationship to God and God's love for humankind. Through revelation, we discover that man is made by God in his own image and likeness. Indeed, it is precisely from this likeness that man's personhood is derived. God "is the most perfect personal Being" and "the whole world of created persons derives its distinctness from and its natural superiority over the world of things (non-persons) from a very particular resemblance to God" (LR, 40). Simultaneously, we discover that God's creative will extends not merely to the human species in general but to each "concrete, unique, and unrepeatable" human being.[54] "Man's coming into being" writes John Paul,

> does not conform to the laws of biology alone, but also, and directly, to God's creative will, which is concerned with the genealogy of the sons and daughters of human families. *God "willed" man from the very beginning, and God "wills" him in every act of conception and every human birth.* God "wills" man as a being similar to himself, as a person. This man, every man, is created by God *"for his own sake."* That is true of all persons, including those born with sicknesses or disabilities.[55]

Indeed, John Paul takes pains to stress that when the Constitution on the Church in the Modern World describes man as "the only creature on earth which God willed for itself," it is speaking not about the species as a whole but about every man, every man not as "part of the multitude of humanity" but each and every particular individual in his or her uniqueness and particularity.[56] At the very center of revelation, however, is found the person of Jesus Christ.

John Paul describes the following passage from the Constitution on the Church in the Modern World as "one of [his] constant references points" (FR, 60, 78): "The truth is that only in the mystery of the incarnate Word does the mystery of man take on light. . . . Christ the New Adam . . . fully reveals man . . . to himself."[57] Through Christ, John Paul writes, God has not only revealed himself fully to mankind, but "has definitively drawn close to it" and has effected its salvation (RM, 11, 31). Through Christ, God has revealed to man "the mystery of the Father and His Love" and "makes man's supreme calling clear."[58] It is thus only in Christ and through Christ that man acquires a "full awareness of his dignity, of the heights to which he is raised, of the surpassing worth of his own humanity, and of the meaning of his existence" (RM, 11, 31).

To begin with, "to the sons of Adam," Christ restores the divine likeness that had been disfigured from the first sin onward.[59] He not only restores our unique dignity,[60] he also raises this dignity to new heights. Here again, John Paul is fond of invoking the Constitution on the Church in the Modern World:

> since human nature as He assumed it was not annulled, by that very fact it has been raised up to a divine dignity in our respect too. For by His incarnation the Son of God has united Himself in some fashion with every man. He worked with human hands, He thought with a human mind, acted by human choice, and loved with a human heart. Born of the Virgin Mary, He truly has been made one of us, like us in all things except sin.[61]

Through the incarnation, God reveals the immensity of his love for humankind.

The exaltation of man's dignity through the incarnation is further accentuated through God's saving action in Christ and the destiny to which man is called by virtue of it. On the one hand, the price of our redemption—Christ's sacrificial death on the cross—is a further proof of the value God himself sets on man and of our dignity in Christ (RM, 20, 81). "How precious must man be in the eyes of the Creator, . . . if God 'gave his only Son' in order that man 'should not perish but have eternal life'" (RM, 10, 28). How precious must man be "if the Son of God pays the supreme price for his dignity."[62]

On the other hand, through Christ, God makes man's supreme calling clear. "In God's plan," John Paul writes, "the vocation of the person extends beyond the boundaries of time."[63] God calls man to eternal life, to the everlasting happiness that comes from union with God, to "the participation in the life of God Himself, which comes about in the eternal communion of the Father, the Son, and the Holy Spirit. . . . In

Jesus Christ, man is called to such a participation and led toward it."[64]
In Jesus Christ, man is offered the grace of divine adoption (RM, 11, 32)
and is summoned to share in God's own divine life.[65]

V

This vision of nature and dignity of the person differs in a number of
important respects from that which has informed the modern quest for
freedom. On the one hand, its metaphysical and moral realism allows
for the existence of an objective and universally binding moral order
accessible to the human mind, an order of human ends which obligates
the conscience prior to, and independently of, our free consent to
strive for them. At the same time, this realism provides a secure grounding for the dignity of the human person. From this perspective, the idea
of human dignity is more than a mere convention, but rather the fundamental ontological fact from which human social and political life
must take its bearings

This dignity has profound implications for the ordering of interpersonal relations. It means that

> A person must not be merely the means to an end for another per-
> son. This is precluded by the very nature of personhood, by what
> any person is. For a person is a thinking subject, and capable of
> taking decision. . . . This being so, every person is by nature capable
> of determining his or her aims. Anyone who treats a person as a
> means to an end does violence to the very essence of the other, to
> what constitutes its natural right. (LR, 26–27)

Nobody—not even God the Creator—can use a person as a means
toward an end, as a mere object to be used to further the ends of another
subject (LR, 27, 28).

"This elementary truth," John Paul concludes, is "an inherent com-
ponent of the natural moral order." Indeed, it finds expression in Kant's
insistence that we must "act always in such a way that the person is the
end and not merely the instrument" of our actions (LR, 41). Although
conveying an extraordinarily important truth, John Paul argues, this
formulation is too negative to do justice to the objective demands of

man's personal dignity. Stated positively, the personalistic norm affirms that "the person is a good towards which the only adequate attitude is love." It is this personalist norm which the commandment to love presupposes and expresses (LR, 41). And, it is this norm that constitutes the basis of all the freedoms proper to the human person, especially freedom of conscience (LR, 28).

At the same time, this vision of the nature and dignity of the human person issues in a different understanding of the nature of freedom from that which dominates contemporary Western culture. To be properly understood, John Paul maintains, human freedom must be seen in the context of "the truth about man" (VS, 87, 107–8). It thus must be seen in the context "of everything which determines the full 'realization' of his humanity."[66]

It is no accident, John Paul insists, that, in the words of the Declaration of Religious Liberty, men are impelled by their nature to seek the truth and to order their whole lives in accord with its demands of truth.[67] Nor is it an accident that we can discern in man "an elemental need of the good, a natural drive and striving towards it" (LR, 29). As persons, human beings are impelled by their nature to realize themselves fully, and thus to be true to their natures (FR, 25, 39). Inasmuch as only true values can enable people to achieve this objective, man's drive toward the perfection of his nature manifests itself in a drive toward truth and goodness. The person, in short, "realizes himself by the exercise of freedom in truth,"[68] through this ordering of his actions, and ultimately his very self, in accordance with the truth.

An adequate account of the requirements of human self-realization, however, cannot limit itself to truth and goodness. Man, John Paul writes, "cannot live without love," he is "incomprehensible" to himself, "his life is senseless" if "he does not experience" love "and make it his own" (RM, 10, 27). The reason for this is found in man's very nature as a being made in the image and likeness of a triune God, a God consisting of three divine persons united in a relation of self-giving love, united in communion. "In speaking of the likeness of God," John Paul writes, "the Second Vatican Council refers not only to the divine image and likeness which every human being as such already possesses, but also and primarily to 'a certain similarity between the union of the divine persons and the union of God's children in truth and love.'"[69] "Human beings," he writes, "are like God not only by reason of their spiritual nature, . . . but also by reason of their capacity for community with other persons" (PC, 318).

By virtue of his likeness to the Trinity, man "who is the only creature on earth which God willed for itself, cannot fully find himself except through a sincere gift of the self."[70] Insofar as the human person can only find fulfillment through the sincere gift of self,[71] it follows that "human perfection . . . consists not simply in acquiring an abstract knowledge of the truth, but in a dynamic relationship of faithful self-giving with others" (FR, 32, 44). Insofar, this is to say, as love is the fundamental and innate vocation of the human person,[72] we can realize ourselves only by entering into relationships "of solidarity and communion with others."[73]

To say that inscribed on the very structure of human nature there exists a natural orientation toward truth, goodness and love, John Paul contends, is to affirm that man experiences "a call to the absolute and transcendent" (FR, 83, 105) and thus a natural (if not always conscious) desire for God. The reason why is not mysterious. "The values by which the person as such lives are by nature transtemporal" and "demand a more complete realization than they find in temporal life. . . . In fact, since these values are themselves absolute, they demand some sort of more complete and definitive realization in the dimensions of the Absolute" (PC, 175). Only God, who is both "the Truth" (VS, 84, 105) and "the Supreme Good" (VS, 98, 120), can satisfy the demands of the human spirit. Insofar, moreover, as God is both "the most perfect personal Being" (LR, 40) and infinite "Love,"[74] it is he "who alone can fully accept our gift" of self,[75] he who alone can satisfy our thirst for communion, for the giving and receiving of love. Thus, John Paul invokes St. Augustine's celebrated formulation that "our heart is restless until it finds its rest in" God.[76] In God man finds "fullness of life, the final end of human activity, and perfect happiness" (VS, 9, 19–20).

Since man possesses a particular bodily and spiritual structure and thus requires certain fundamental goods as the condition of his self-realization, it follows that human nature cannot be reduced to a freedom which is self-designing (VS, 48, 66). An adequate account of human nature must understand freedom in the light of its essential and constitutive relationship to truth (VS, 4, 13). God, John Paul writes, "left man 'in the power of his own counsel' (Sir 15, 14), that he might freely seek his Creator and freely attain perfection. Attaining such

perfection means personally building up that perfection in himself"
(VS, 39, 55).

"Human freedom," writes John Paul, "belongs to us as creatures; it
is a freedom which is given as a gift, one to be received like a seed and
to be cultivated responsibly. It is an essential part of the creaturely image
which is the basis of the dignity of the person." Accordingly, this freedom is not absolute and unconditional, but limited and finite. "At once
inalienable self-possession and openness to all that exists," it is ordered
to truth, goodness, and love (VS, 87, 107–8) because it is only through
these goods that freedom can achieve its purpose of enabling people
to realize themselves fully by being true to their nature (FR, 25, 39)
and fulfilling the destiny to which they are called by their Creator.
Human freedom, therefore, is "realized through the willing and choosing of a true Good" (PC, 234).

If in order to effectively seek his Creator and his perfection man
must freely do good and avoid evil, this means that he must be able to
distinguish good from evil (VS, 42, 58). This discernment comes about
through man's reason, in particular by his reason enlightened by Divine
Revelation and by faith (VS, 44, 60). God, this is to say,

> provides for man differently from the way he provides for beings
> which are not persons. He cares for man not "from without,"
> through laws of physical nature, but "from within," through reason,
> which, by its natural knowledge of God's eternal law, is conse-
> quently able to show man the right direction to take in his free
> actions. In this way God calls man to participate in his own provi-
> dence. (VS, 43, 59)

Inasmuch as "God, who alone is good, knows perfectly what is good
for man" and "by virtue of his very love proposes this good to man"
through the moral law, it follows that "human freedom finds its complete and authentic fulfillment precisely in the acceptance" of this law.
"God's law does not reduce, much less do away with human freedom,"
but instead protects and promotes that freedom (VS, 35, 51) because by
submitting to it "freedom submits to the truth of creation," to "the
requirements and the promptings" of "divine wisdom" (VS, 41, 56).
Since "the good of the person is to be in the Truth and to *do* the Truth"
(VS, 84, 105), it is only through obedience to God's law (VS, 41, 56) that

human freedom can achieve its goal of enabling human persons to realize themselves fully.

Obedience to God therefore is not contrary to the dignity of the person because it does not represent "a heteronomy, as if the moral life were subject to the will of something all powerful, absolute, extraneous to man and intolerant of his freedom." On the contrary, human freedom and God's law meet in man's free obedience to God and God's completely gratuitous benevolence toward man. "Since man's free obedience to God's law effectively implies that human will participates in God's wisdom and providence," this obedience must be seen as a *"participated* theonomy" (VS, 41, 56–57). Insofar as human freedom is ordered to the perfection of the human person and God's law embodies the demands of the goods whereby this perfection is attained, this law "expresses the dignity of the person" (BS, 51, 69). Thus, it is only through obedience to the law that human freedom conforms to human dignity (VS, 42, 58). Indeed, to obey this law is man's very dignity (VS, 53, 73).

Human freedom, therefore, is not unlimited. When man rejects the moral law given by God (VS, 35, 50), the result is "the death of true freedom: 'Truly, truly, I say to you, every one who commits sin is a slave to sin' (Jn 8:34)" (EV, 20, 39). For this reason, authentic freedom is "never freedom 'from' the truth but always and only freedom 'in' the truth" (VS, 64, 82). Freedom therefore "does not realize itself in decisions made against God. For how could it be an exercise of true freedom to refuse to be open to the very reality which enables our self-realization?" (FR, 13, 23).

Precisely because freedom has its foundation and finds its complete and authentic fulfillment (VS, 35, 51) in the truth, there can be no freedom apart from or in opposition to truth (VS, 96, 118). Thus, "far from being a limitation upon freedom or a threat to it," John Paul writes, "reference to the truth about the human person—a truth universally knowable through the moral law written through the hearts of all—is, in fact, the guarantor of freedom's future."[77]

VI

Several years ago, John Paul told a group of American bishops that in rejecting today's pervasive "skepticism regarding the existence of 'moral truth' and an objective moral law," and affirming the essential bond between freedom and truth,

> you will be challenging one of the great forces in the modern world. But at the same time, *you will be doing the modern world a great service,* for you will be reminding it of the only foundation capable of sustaining a culture of freedom: what the Founders of your nation called "self-evident" truths.[78]

The great service he asks them to perform consists in helping to save modernity from itself by helping to rescue one of the noblest aspirations of the modern era—the quest for freedom—from the currents within modernity itself that threaten it. This threat issues from the very metaphysics of the person through which modern thought has conceptualized human freedom and dignity of their demands. Insofar as it leads freedom to detach itself from truth, this metaphysics causes the modern quest for freedom to negate and destroy itself.

If he rejects modernity's metaphysics of the person, John Paul rejects neither modernity as such nor the exaltation of freedom it has engendered. On the contrary, he affirms that modernity's aspiration to achieve *"the complete liberation of man"* is a "noble" one.[79] Likewise, he embraces the quest for freedom which this aspiration has prompted in political life, insisting that respect for the dignity of the human person necessarily entails a commitment to the protection and promotion of freedom. He advocates neither a retreat to the premodern past nor the embrace of some new type of authoritarian political order. Rather, insisting that "freedom is the measure of man's dignity and greatness" and that the great challenge confronting us "today is the responsible use of freedom, in both its personal and social dimensions,"[80] he calls on us to carry the modern quest for freedom through to a successful conclusion. To do so will require correcting and purifying it in the light of "the whole truth about man" and thus of "the truth and love revealed to men by Jesus Christ."[81]

Notes

Support for this article comes in part from a grant from The Pew Charitable Trusts. The opinions expressed in this essay are those of the author and do not necessarily reflect the views of The Pew Charitable Trusts. In citing papal and conciliar documents, the section number is given followed by the page number in the edition being cited.

1. Walter Kasper, *The Christian Understanding of Freedom and the History of Freedom in the Modern Era: The Meeting and Confrontation between Christianity and the Modern Era in a Postmodern Situation*, 1988 Père Marquette Lecture in Theology (Milwaukee: Marquette University Press, 1988), 12–13.

2. See Charles Taylor, *The Ethics of Authenticity* (Cambridge: Harvard University Press, 1991), 13–24.

3. Kenneth L. Schmitz, *At the Center of the Human Drama: The Philosophical Anthropology of Karol Wojtyla/Pope John Paul II* (Washington, D.C.: Catholic University of America Press, 1993), 122.

4. *On the Relationship between Faith and Reason [Fides et Ratio]* (Boston: St. Paul Books and Media, 1998), [section] 84, [p.] 107. Hereafter, this document will be cited parenthetically as FR.

5. *The Redeemer of Man [Redemptor Hominis]* (Washington, D.C.: United States Catholic Conference, 1979), 17, 60. Hereafter, this document will be cited parenthetically as RM.

6. "Homily at a Mass in Aqueduct Racetrack, Queens, New York, October 6, 1995," in *Make Room for the Mystery of God: Visit of Pope John Paul II to the USA 1995* (Boston: St. Paul Books and Media, 1995), 51.

7. Quoted in Henri de Lubac, *At the Service of the Church* (San Francisco: Ignatius Press, 1993), 171.

8. George Weigel, *Witness to Hope: The Biography of Pope John Paul II* (New York: Harper Collins, 1999).

9. "Homily at a Mass in Aqueduct Racetrack," 51.

10. Quoted in de Lubac, *At the Service of the Church*, 172.

11. "Homily at a Mass in Aqueduct Racetrack," 51.

12. Quoted in de Lubac, *At the Service of the Church*, 172.

13. *Declaration on Religious Freedom (Dignitatis Humanae)*, in *The Sixteen Documents of Vatican II* (Boston: Pauline Books and Media, 1999), 1, 491.

14. *On Social Concern [Sollicitudo Rei Socialis]* (Boston: St. Paul Books and Media, n.d. [1987]).

15. *The Splendor of Truth [Veritatis Splendor]* (Boston: St. Paul Books & Media, n.d. [1993]), 31, 45. Hereafter, this document will be cited parenthetically as VS.

16. Karol Wojtyla [Pope John Paul II], *Person and Community: Selected Essays*, trans. Theresa Sandak, O.S.M. (New York: Peter Lang, 1993), 220. Hereafter, this work will be cited parenthetically as PC. Since our interest here is the thought of Pope John Paul II, we will rely primarily on his encyclicals and official pronouncements. We will, however, draw on his earlier works when they assist us in understanding the vision that animates these documents.

17. John Paul II, *The Gospel of Life* [*Evangelim Vitae*] (Boston: St. Paul Books & Media, n.d. [1995]), 25, 46. Hereafter, this document will be cited parenthetically as EV.

18. "Address to the General Assembly of the United Nations," October 5, 1995, in *Make Room for the Mystery of God: Visit of John Paul II to the USA 1995* (Boston: Pauline Books & Media, 1995), 21.

19. *Pastoral Constitution on the Church in the Modern World* [*Gaudium et Spes*], in *The Sixteen Documents of Vatican II*, 17, 214.

20. "Address to the General Assembly," 21, 19.

21. *Pastoral Constitution on the Church in the Modern World*, 17, 639.

22. Karol Wojtyla, *Love and Responsibility* (San Francisco: Ignatius Press, 1993), 24. Hereafter, this work will be cited parenthetically as LR.

23. *Pastoral Constitution on the Church in the Modern World*, 17, 214.

24. Ibid.

25. *Crossing the Threshold of Hope*, ed. Vittorio Messori (New York: Alfred A. Knopf, 1994), 196.

26. *On the Hundredth Anniversary of Rerum Novarum* [*Centesimus Annus*] (Boston: St. Paul Books & Media, n.d. [1991]), 44, 64.

27. "Freedom and the Moral Law," in *Springtime of Evangelization: The Complete Texts of the Holy Father's 1998 Ad Limina Addresses to the Bishops of the United States*, ed. Thomas D. Williams, L.C. (San Diego: Basilica Press, 1999), 5, 117.

28. *On Social Concern*, 26, 42.

29. "Address to the General Assembly," 20.

30. Quoted in *New York Times*, April 6, 1987. Cited in George Weigel, *Freedom and Its Discontents* (Washington, D.C.: Ethics and Public Policy Center, 1991), 45.

31. *On Social Concern*, 44, 84.

32. Quoted in *New York Times*, April 6, 1987. Cited in Weigel, *Freedom and Its Discontents*, 45.

33. See, for example, "John Paul on the American Experiment," *First Things*, no. 82 (April 1998): 36–37. This article consists of the text of John Paul's remarks on receiving the credentials of the Honorable Lindy Boggs as ambassador to the Holy See on December 16, 1997.

34. *On the Hundredth Anniversary*, 46, 65.

35. "Freedom and the Moral Law," 5, 117; 6, 118.

36. *On the Hundredth Anniversary*, 44, 64.

37. "Freedom and the Moral Law," 6, 118.

38. *On the Hundredth Anniversary*, 46, 65.

39. "Freedom and the Moral Law," 6, 118.

40. Ibid., 2, 112.

41. Ibid., 2, 111–12.

42. Ibid., 2, 111.

43. *On the Hundredth Anniversary*, 44, 64–65; 45, 65.

44. "Freedom and the Moral Law," 2, 111–12.

45. Ibid., 111.

46. *On the Hundredth Anniversary*, 11, 18.

47. For good overviews of John Paul's thought, see Schmitz, *At the Center of the Human Drama;* Weigel, *Witness to Hope;* Rocco Buttiglione, *Karol Wojtyla: The Thought of the Man Who Became Pope John Paul II* (Grand Rapids, Mich.: William B. Eerdmans, 1997); George H. Williams, *The Mind of Pope John Paul II: Origins of His Thought and Action* (New York: Seabury, 1981); and Avery Dulles, *The Splendor of Faith: The Theological Vision of Pope John Paul II* (New York: Crossroad, 1999).

48. John F. Crosby, *The Selfhood of the Human Person* (Washington, D.C.: Catholic University Press of America, 1996), 4, 82.

49. *Declaration on Religious Freedom*, 2, 679.

50. "Homily of a Mass in Central Park, New York City, October 7, 1995," in *Make Room for the Mystery of God*, 65.

51. Ibid.

52. Cited in *Human Rights in the Teaching Church: From John XXIII to John Paul II*, ed. Giorgio Filibeck (Vatican City: Libreria Editrice Vaticana, 1994), 51. The remarks cited were originally contained in a speech delivered by John Paul in 1984 ("Address to the General Audience," 25 January 1984).

53. *Pastoral Constitution on the Church in the Modern World*, 24, 233.

54. *Letter to Families from Pope John Paul II* (Boston: St. Paul Books & Media, 1994), 11, 31.

55. Ibid., 9, 22.

56. Ibid., 9, 22, and 11, 31.

57. *Pastoral Constitution on the Church in the Modern World*, 22, 220.

58. Ibid.

59. Ibid.

60. *Crossing the Threshold of Hope*, 17.

61. *Pastoral Constitution on the Church in the Modern World*, 22, 221.

62. *Crossing the Threshold of Hope*, 197.

63. *Letter to Families*, 9, 23.

64. *Crossing the Threshold of Hope*, 71–72.

65. *Letter to Families*, 9, 23.

66. Ibid., 14, 46.

67. *Declaration on Religious Freedom*, 2, 679.

68. *Letter to Families*, 14, 45.

69. *Letter to Families*, 8, 19.

70. *Pastoral Constitution on the Church in the Modern World*, 24, 223.

71. *Letter to Families,* 11, 28.

72. *The Role of the Christian Family in the Modern World* [*Familiaris Consortio*] (Boston: St. Paul Editions, n.d. [1981]), 11, 22.

73. *On the Hundredth Anniversary,* 41, 58.

74. *Crossing the Threshold of Hope,* 222.

75. Ibid., 41, 59.

76. *Letter to Families,* 9, 23.

77. "Address to the General Assembly," 30.

78. "Freedom and the Moral Law," 2, 11; 6, 119; 4, 116, my emphasis.

79. "God's Self-Revelation to Humanity," in *Springtime of Evangelization,* 6, 43.

80. "Address to the General Assembly," 30.

81. "God's Self-Revelation to Humanity," 6, 43.

AFTERWORD

Facets of Personal Dignity

GLENN TINDER

The preceding essays are all occasioned by the strange moral ambiguity of our age. On the one hand, we have seen startling displays of disdain for the human person, sometimes in mad transports of class or racial hatred, sometimes merely in coarse processes of utilitarian reasoning in the single-minded pursuit of profit and power. In the Soviet Gulag and the Nazi death camps the very idea of personal dignity was exultantly trampled upon; more recently, and nearer at hand, arguments for euthanasia or unrestricted abortion rights often have resolutely ignored implicit moral issues and obscured those issues with a depersonalized vocabulary. Respectable and richly rewarded tobacco executives have directed decades-long advertising campaigns which they knew would bring multitudinous deaths; and numerous network executives and film producers have persistently offered entertainment that glamorously defies conventional standards such as the evil of violence and the sanctity of marriage. Future generations will surely be appalled when they look back on some of the things done and suffered in our time.

On the other hand, the "dignity of the individual"—the idea that a human being deserves special concern and is not to be treated merely as something usable or disposable—has apparently become the central maxim of the modern moral creed. This idea is among the most significant insights reached by civilized humanity. It emerged perhaps two thousand years ago, among both Greek philosophers and early Christians. In our time, it has not been forgotten, in spite of being frequently and egregiously violated. On the contrary, it has come to be grounded, at least in many societies, in a firm and broad consensus—a fact sensitively examined by David Walsh's essay. Indeed, the idea has been weakened less by counterarguments than by being so invariably honored in speech that it is now cliché.

It is tempting to say, in view of the glaring contrast between speech and practice, that all of our talk about human dignity is mere hypocrisy. But clearly it is not. People in the twenty-first century, in many quarters at any rate, are almost obsessively concerned with the needs and sensitivities of persons particularly disadvantaged—racial minorities, women, the handicapped, and others who in the past were routinely ignored or suppressed. The dignity of the individual is a cliché, yet it retains surprising force. Future generations perhaps will not despise us altogether.

Still, a firm consensus, however benign, can be a dangerous thing. It may conceal questions which ought to be asked. As the essays in this volume suggest, such is the case with the consensus concerning human dignity. To begin with, have we overemphasized the idea? Even if a human being does possess a peculiar dignity, it could be that exclusive attention to this single moral fact blinds us to other moral facts. It may blind us, for example, to ways in which human beings are unequal, thereby rendering us insensitive to values, such as strength of characters or depth of intellect, which are not equally manifest in everyone. Something of this sort is suggested in Robert Kraynak's essay. Or it might blind us to human needs and sufferings which demand compassion more than they do respect. Timothy Jackson's essay calls attention to a quality in humans which requires that we not merely respect them but respond to their needs. In effect, the Kraynak and Jackson essays compel us to wonder whether by turning a moral insight into a cliché we have in some ways damaged our moral discernment.

Another quite radical question is this: assuming that human beings do possess a peculiar dignity, why is this so? What is it about a human being that demands respect? Why has the idea of the dignity of the individual proven so tenacious? As the essays in this volume show, while there may be a consensus concerning the dignity of persons, there is no consensus concerning the source of that dignity. A human being differs from other creatures in several ways, and each of these ways seems to afford a possible basis for claiming respect. For example, only human beings among earthly creatures possess reason. Is it reason, then, that commands respect? If so, however, why should we respect people who behave unreasonably? And why should we affirm the dignity of the retarded, people deficient in the very power of reason?

Closely associated with reason is a no less mysterious power, that of choosing freely. Unlike any other animal, a human being is compelled continually to decide what to do and what sort of person to be. In Jean-Paul Sartre's famous phrase, one is "condemned to be free." As a common way of speaking has it, a human being is not just a "thing," moved to and fro by causal laws but rather, unlike anything else in the world, is engaged ceaselessly and inescapably in the task of self-direction and thereby of self-creation. Is this a source of dignity? It seems plausible to think that it is. Yet how can we answer someone who asks whether those who most of the time forget their freedom, along with the fact that they are continually shaping their own identities, thus lose their dignity. If they do, it may seem, considering the large part habit and routine play in most lives, that dignity can be claimed only by an exceptional morality.

We face a cognate question if we ask whether our dignity derives from what is sometimes called our "transcendence." This is our ability to stand above and survey every situation in which we find ourselves, and in this way to take cognizance of alternative possibilities of action. The power of transcendence is the power of knowing broad ranges of reality. Certain philosophers, such as Thomas Aquinas and Immanuel Kant, brought out the fact that by virtue of this power the human mind is, as it were, a miniature universe, a microcosmos. A human being is not merely one among the countless creatures dwelling within the universe. The universe is in a certain fashion within each human being—a condition powerfully suggestive of dignity.

A like condition was emphasized by a philosopher heavily influenced by Kant, G. W. F. Hegel. Hegel was particularly impressed by the capacity of human beings to comprehend (with the guidance of philosophers) the emergence of their own humanity in history. From Hegel's perspective a person is a miniature version not only of the cosmos, in all of its vast impersonality, but of the whole drama of human life on earth. And since that drama is not something accidental and alien, according to Hegel, but in essence is the logical unfolding of the human mind and spirit, a person is lifted up and in some sense sanctified by comprehending human history. In contemplating the destiny of the human race, an individual discovers the grand outlines of his own personal dignity. This idea was at the core of the book *Against Fate: An Essay on Personal Dignity,* which occasioned the present volume.

Transcendence is a dramatic power. It apparently marks off human beings sharply from all other entities. But how many people evince that power? How many possess anything but a very sketchy, and even partially false, conception of the universe and of human history? Surely very few. But if transcendence is the source of our dignity, and transcendence is realized in microcosmic and microhistorical breadth, doesn't it follow that possessors of dignity make up only a tiny elite? Such a conclusion would be very distant from the meaning that "the dignity of the individual" has from the beginning conveyed to most minds: that dignity belongs somehow to every person.

Reason, freedom, transcendence, and microcosmic breadth all imply a kind of exaltation. It is this exaltation, seemingly, that gives rise to the idea of human dignity. In contrast, one of the most time-honored and potent concepts of human dignity derives from an idea that implies subjection; this is the idea that men and women are the only creatures who can place themselves under a moral law. In other words, they are the only creatures capable of righteousness. It is arguable that some of the earliest appearances of the idea of human dignity, among Stoic philosophers of the Hellenistic and Roman eras, occurred in response to such an insight. And certainly the most powerful modern affirmation of human dignity, that found in the moral philosophy of Kant, arose from a sense of the human capacity for righteousness. (To be accurate, however, we must note that subjection to the moral law was seen by Kant as paradoxically a kind of exaltation; every person is able to formulate the moral law and thereby to stand as a kind of legislator for the entire human race.) Kant's moral outlook, and the vision of human dignity that followed from it—memorably expressed in the imperative that you must treat humankind, both in yourself and in every other person, always "as an end, never merely as a means"—are expertly brought to light in Susan Shell's essay.

Like all theories of human dignity, however, this particular theory involves some difficult questions. One such question is whether only the righteous are possessors of dignity. If so, it might be asked whether the unrighteous, those who have committed serious offenses, have forfeited every claim to respect. If they have, can we then justifiably subject them to any punishments, however brutal, that are calculated to discourage further offenses? Or can a society, in good conscience, simply eliminate them? The idea of human dignity surely is greatly diluted if it allows for such inferences as these. A noteworthy aspect of Western judicial systems is that even those convicted of the most serious crimes retain many rights and are normally treated with painstaking care.

A question of a very different sort about the derivation of human dignity from moral capacity is often raised today in college classrooms. Doesn't the claim to be righteous, or even to know what righteousness is, inevitably lead to intolerance and in that way to a denial of the dignity of those judged to be unrighteous? Moral relativism—the conviction that morality is relative to time and place, and thus is not the same for everyone—is widespread in American universities, and it gives rise to one of the most significant questions we face today. Does such relativism undergird a "live-and-let-live" attitude which grants everyone, whether their neighbors approve of them or not, a degree of respect? Or does it subtly trivialize human beings, treating them as nothing more than complex animals, hence subject, when necessity dictates, to being treated like animals—merely as means, and not as ends in themselves?

Allied with the idea that our dignity depends on submitting to the moral law is that it depends on our submitting to God. Human beings are often distinctly inglorious. If there is no God to serve as a bestower of glory, can we attribute dignity—presumably a kind of glory—to every human being? In Western culture, as Robert Kraynak brings out, the notion of personal dignity has been closely connected with the great biblical theme that men and women are created in "the image and likeness of God." A human being is not merely a microcosmos but is a microtheos. Dignity was bestowed in the act of divine creation. In Christian narrative this dignity was forfeited in the course of a great rebellion against God, often called "original sin." It is restored, however, in the act of divine redemption that occurred in the crucifixion and resurrection of Christ. In that event, the whole human race was judged, punished, and raised up into a new life. In modern times, however, we are apparently witnessing the spread of religious skepticism. What does this mean for human dignity? Do agnosticism and atheism, by denying creation and divine redemption, implicitly degrade the human species? Is a religious skeptic an incipient nihilist?

All of these questions, let us remember, are reducible to one we started with: What is it about a person that inspires respect, even in an age that often seems respectful of nothing? Questions of a different kind, however, are suggested by some of the essays in this volume. These concern the implications of personal dignity for the social and political order. How can the dignity of individuals be adequately recognized and safeguarded by society? For example, does personal dignity imply personal liberty? It is noteworthy that the two great Christians discussed in this volume, Martin Luther (whose dramatic vision of human freedom is masterfully described by John Witte, Jr.) and Pope John Paul II (whose political thought is comprehensively laid out in Kenneth Grasso's essay) agree that the capacity for choice enters into the dignity of persons; they agree too that such dignity comes ultimately from God. But they agree not at all on what these things mean for society and polity. For the pope, as for many others today, personal dignity points toward the ideal of societies in which all are free to shape their own lives. In a word, dignity implies democracy. Luther, on the other hand, saw human beings as wicked in spite of their dignity (which derived from their faith, not their actual conduct) and thus as needing strong, authoritarian rule. Such rule was not necessarily incompatible with their dignity. For Luther, the sacredness of the individual, although defined in terms of inward freedom, implied little in the way of outward freedom.

Even those who agree on the need for outward freedom, however, often disagree concerning the nature of such freedom. Does it imply a right to think and speak and live altogether as one pleases, or can it be realized in a settled and specific social role—the kind of role spoken of by a modern philosopher as one's "station and its duties"? For many, to speak of a broad range of individual rights is to speak in the most adequate way possible of the institutional meaning of the dignity of the individual. This is the attitude we usually call "liberalism." But for many present-day scholars and thinkers, including the pope, the liberal emphasis on individual rights arouses serious misgivings. It smacks too much of self-interest and says far too little about obligations toward others. It is connected, moreover, with an individualism which is oblivious of all the ties that render a human being dependent on society, not merely for a satisfactory life from day to day, but for the very qualities that render one human. Freedom, in the minds of these critics, is enjoyed only in a life of social and civic activity. It is defined less by rights than by duties.

If liberty is the first great institutional ideal of the modern world, equality is the second. What does personal dignity say about equality? Are human beings, as we often benevolently but thoughtlessly assume, really equal in dignity? Were all the laborers who helped Michelangelo deal with the huge stones he sculpted equal in dignity to Michelangelo himself? Was every Briton alive in wartime England equal in dignity to Winston Churchill? In asking these questions we return to the hierarchical world sketched out in Robert Kraynak's essay. It is somewhat surprising that the notion of equality has gained so powerful a hold on the human mind, for equality is far from a conspicuous characteristic of the world around us. Reality in general, ranged in ranks ascending from inorganic matter to plants and trees, and thence to irrational animals, and thence to humans, with their powers of reason, choice, and transcendence—and ascending thence, in many minds, to angels and to God—is quite definitely, even splendidly, hierarchical. Also hierarchical is humanity within itself. It is hard to think of a single significant human quality—courage, beauty, health, agility, learning, wisdom, righteousness—which is not quite unequally possessed. By virtue of what quality are human beings equal? If by none, how can human equality be affirmed without threatening our very awareness of the virtues and values which render that universe meaningful and human life worthwhile?

Yet how can such inequalities be recognized in the social order? Are we able to build meritocracies so exact that social and natural inequalities correspond? It is hard to think so, given the chaos and injustice prevailing in most societies today; as examples of human statecraft, these seem to demonstrate gross ineptitude. Someone might claim that even though the realms of nature and humanity are sharply hierarchical, it is better that we treat one another as if we were equal. Blinded as we are by prejudice and ignorance, we are poor judges of human excellence. Further, even if we were very good judges of human excellence, we would be very poor distributors of wealth and power and honor. Not only are we ordinarily clumsy in our organizational efforts; we are proud and selfish to a degree that causes us invariably to favor ourselves and our friends. There is safety, therefore, only in the rule of equality. And aside from the matter of practicality, there is the matter of personal dignity. Every individual can presumably claim at least a minute measure of worth. An egalitarian social order would not be entirely unjust. Indeed, John Rawls has constructed a highly influential argument showing that equality is the very essence of justice and the foundation of a well-ordered society.

Such an argument has a look of good sense. Yet, its limitations are plain to most people today, and even Rawls acknowledges those limitations. While it is difficult to distribute riches, offices, and privileges in accordance with a hierarchy of excellence, it is no less difficult to distribute them with perfect equality. The effort has invariably failed. And when the effort has been applied in deadly earnestness, it has given rise to extreme and violent inequalities (remember Pol Pot). Moreover, trying to establish complete equality would require us to blind ourselves morally. Divesting ourselves of the ability to discriminate among values and persons, and doing this at the behest of an abstract principle like equality, is hardly a promising preparation for the task of ordering our lives in common.

In sum, the standards of equality and hierarchy both have strong claims on us; neither, at the same time, seems practicable. Here, however, an objection may be raised. The human race, someone might argue, is not in such a quandary as my comments suggest. Corresponding to the consensus concerning the dignity of the human person is a consensus concerning the political and economic order that best recognizes and safeguards this dignity. The ideal of liberal democracy, that is, of government that is legally limited and based on popular consent, has come to be almost universally accepted (even though far from universally practiced). And the assumption that liberal democracy is properly accompanied by a market economy, in some degree tempered by considerations of justice and need, is granted almost everywhere. It has even been argued that we are approaching "the end of history," which seems true at least in the sense that no one can see in what direction the human race might proceed once it has realized these apparently quite realizable ideals.

The force of this objection must be granted; we are not utterly overwhelmed by uncertainties. It is tempting, however, to liken the certainties we seemingly possess—concerning the dignity of persons and the desirability of liberal, democratic, and capitalist institutions—to redoubts behind which we fight to save a declining civilization. Outside these redoubts there is profound confusion. While liberal democracy and capitalism may be widely accepted, these seem to allow or even call forth conditions like an obsession with money, a coarse popular culture, and drastic economic inequalities—conditions alarming enough to create widespread doubts about the health of our civilization.

Moreover, while our certitudes may be impressive, they are dangerously disconnected from any general structure of fealties and beliefs. Our situation would be less alarming were we sustained by strong religious and philosophical convictions. But we are not. This is shown by the secularism and religious skepticism seemingly rife among the most highly educated groups in modern society. It is shown too by the power of the deconstructionist movement (or "postmodernism") among Western intellectuals. Pontius Pilate is often thought of as profoundly cynical for having asked at Jesus' trial, "What is truth?" But Pilate may have assumed that such a thing as truth existed. Today numerous literate and philosophical people have called any such assumption into question. Their response to Pilate is that truth is whatever powerful people are inclined to believe and are able to get others to believe.

What then must we do? At the very least, it seems, we must think. Thinking is a way of standing within our redoubts and fighting for civilized values. One of the most promising features of our situation—in so many ways ominous—is that the idea of personal dignity is apparently a powerful stimulus to thought. Thus David Walsh's essay suggests that reflecting on that idea may enable us to delve into the metaphysical depths that seem in our time so impenetrable. The other essays in this volume demonstrate the validity of this suggestion. Not that they give us a single answer to the question of the source and the institutional meaning of personal dignity, or even that the diverse answers they provide fit neatly together. Rather, they show us that the idea of personal dignity is not a simple principle, plain in its meaning, which we can learn and use as we do the principles governing the operation of our automobiles and computers. It is a mystery, a matter of reflection and meditation, and on occasion, perhaps, a matter of public dialogue. It is like a cut and polished diamond, facets of which the essays in this volume display. So long as we are discerning and serious enough frequently to contemplate this gem, surely our situation is far from desperate.

CONTRIBUTORS

Kenneth L. Grasso is professor of political science at Southwest Texas State University in San Marcos, Texas. He is the coeditor of *John Courtney Murray and the American Civil Conversation* and *Catholicism, Liberalism, and Communitarianism: The Catholic Intellectual Tradition and the Moral Foundations of Democracy.*

Timothy P. Jackson is associate professor of Christian ethics in the Candler School of Theology at Emory University in Atlanta, Georgia. He is the author of *Love Disconsoled: Meditations on Christian Charity* and *The Priority of Love: Christian Charity and Social Justice.*

Robert P. Kraynak is professor of political science at Colgate University in Hamilton, New York. He is the author of *History and Modernity in the Thought of Thomas Hobbes* and, most recently, *Christian Faith and Modern Democracy.*

John Rawls is professor of philosophy, emeritus, at Harvard University. He is the author of *A Theory of Justice, Political Liberalism,* and *The Law of Peoples.*

Susan M. Shell is professor of political science at Boston College in Chestnut Hill, Massachusetts. She is the author of *The Rights of Reason: A Study of Kant's Philosophy and Politics; The Embodiment of Reason: Kant on Spirit, Generation, and Community;* and articles on Machiavelli, Rousseau, German Idealism, and American political thought.

Glenn Tinder is professor of political science, emeritus, at the University of Massachusetts in Boston. He is the author of many works of political philosophy and theology, including *Political Thinking; Against Fate: An Essay on Personal Dignity; The Political Meaning of Christianity;* and *The Fabric of Hope.*

David Walsh is professor of politics at The Catholic University of America in Washington, D.C. He is the author of *After Ideology: Recovering the Spiritual Foundations of Freedom; The Growth of the Liberal Soul; The Third Millennium: Reflections on Faith and Reason;* and *Guarded by Mystery: Meaning in a Postmodern Age.*

John Witte, Jr., is the Jonas Robitscher Professor of Law and Ethics, director of the Law and Religion Program, and director of the Center for the Interdisciplinary Study of Religion at Emory University School of Law in Atlanta, Georgia. He has published numerous articles and books, including *From Sacrament to Contract: Marriage, Religion, and Law in the Western Tradition; Proselytism and Orthodoxy in Russia; Religion and the American Constitutional Experiment;* and most recently, *Law and Protestantism: The Legal Teachings of the Lutheran Reformation.*

Abel and Cain (OT figures), 130–31
abortion, 141
    and *Roe v. Wade*, 141–42, 152–53
Abraham (OT figure), 86, 125
Acropolis (Athenian), 40
Adam and Eve (OT figures), 29,
    84–85, 130–31
agnosticism, 188
Alzheimer's disease, 150, 159
angels, 99–101
Aquinas, Saint Thomas, 53, 98–104,
    110, 239
Aristotle, 28, 38, 53, 62–63, 81,
    96–98, 221
assisted suicide, 141, 152
Augustine, Saint, 23, 34, 96,
    99–101, 229
autonomy, 55–58, 71, 113, 143, 159,
    163n.34, 180, 200, 216

Barth, Karl, 33
Becket, Thomas, 35
Bergson, Henri, 31
Bishop, Elizabeth, 47
Buber, Martin, 33, 111
Buddhism, 154, 156

Caesar, Julius, 35
Calvin, John, and Calvinism, 103, 106
Carter, Jimmy, 105
Cassuto, Umberto, 85
Christianity, 12, 29
    and democracy, 105–12
    and hierarchy, 114–15, 116n.10
    Kantian influence on, 108–12

    and natural universe, 39, 113
    and sanctity, 142
    transcendent view of the person,
        170–73, 187
    view of human dignity, 81–115
    view of original sin, 21, 241
    Voegelin's view, 103–5
Churchill, Sir Winston, 243
Copernicus, 5

Darwin, Charles, 5
Declaration of Independence, 131, 181
democracy, 106–12, 139
    ascendency in West, 139
    complementary to Christianity,
        105–6
    John Paul II's view, 214–15
    and mass society, 2–3
    Protestant influence on, 129–34
    Rorty's view, 167
Descartes, René, 1, 4
destiny
    irony of, 29–33
    as realizing authentic self, 23–29, 111
    as receptivity to transcendence,
        33–36
    Tinder's view, 23–36
Dignitatis Humanae ("Declaration on
    Religious Freedom," Vatican II
    document), 119–20, 125, 210, 228
divine image in man (*Imago Dei*), 7,
    81–115, 186, 216
Dostoevsky, Fyodor, 18–19, 42–44
Dworkin, Ronald, 7
    critique of, 145–53

Eliot, T. S., 41
embryo research, 152
environmentalism, 4, 41, 113
Epicureanism, 46–47
euthanasia, 141–42

fate
  and death, 41–43
  and industrial society,
    36–39
  irony of, 14–16
  Tinder's definition,
    11–12

Greek *polis*, 39–40, 46
Gregory of Nyssa, Saint, 224
Guevara, Che, 32

Hegel, G. W. F., and Hegelianism,
    107, 239
Hitler, Adolf, 15, 18, 44,
    119
Hobbes, Thomas, 55, 66
holiness, 88–89
Hooker, Richard, 106
human dignity
  in Bible, 83–96
  distinguished from sanctity,
    139–60
  and divine election, 113
  hierarchical vs. democratic
    conceptions, 90–91, 115
  of the individual, 11, 28
  Kantian conception, 53–74
  medieval view, 96–105
  in modern theology,
    105–12
  problems in defining and limiting,
    9, 140
  as related to human species, 4–5,
    47–48, 148

root words, *dignitas* and *Würde*,
    53–54, 58
  threats to in our times, 2–6
human rights, 109–10, 120–23, 133,
    165, 181–83

Imago Dei (image of God). *See*
    divine image in man
Islam, 81, 122

Jaspers, Karl, 33, 34
Jesus Christ, 21, 29, 31, 35, 45, 52, 54,
    80n.53, 81, 89, 93–94, 108, 126,
    170, 225–26, 232
Job (OT figure), 39
John XXIII (pope), 110,106, 110
John Paul II (pope), 8, 83, 110, 242
  and modern freedom, 209–16
  and personalism, 210, 222
  and rights and dignity of the
    human person, 83, 212–14
  on Second Vatican Council,
    210–11
  synthesis of Thomism and
    Kantian ideas, 110
  on uniqueness of every human
    being, 221–24
Judaism, 31, 39, 43, 81, 122

Kant, Immanuel, 11, 37, 172, 227, 240
  agnostic toward God, 34
  democratizes concept of human
    dignity, 53–71
  influence on Christianity, 107–15
  influence on John Paul II's
    personalism, 227–28
  influence on Tinder, 11
  and liberalism, 103, 109
Kennedy, John F., 26
King, Martin Luther, 111
Koestler, Arthur, 63

Las Casas, Bartolome de, 107
Lawrence, D. H., 24
Leo XIII (pope), 106
liberalism
    dependence on spiritual
        traditions, 174–75
    and human dignity, 165–88, 242
    Kantian school of, 108–9
    possible roots in Aquinas, 102
    as residual Christianity, 187
Lincoln, Abraham, 7, 28, 49, 139, 157
Locke, John, 55, 150, 168–69, 176, 179
Lubac, Henri de, 209
Luther, Martin, 26, 106, 242
    Freedom of a Christian, 123–34
    and Peasant Revolt of 1525, 129
    on sanctity and depravity, 125

MacIntyre, Alasdair, 178
Mao Tse-tung, 44
Marcel, Gabriel, 109
Maritain, Jacques, 107, 109
Marx, Karl, and Marxism, 32, 36
Michelangelo, 243
Mill, John Stuart, 177, 179
Mirandola, Pico della, *Oration on the
    Dignity of Man*, 6, 54
Murray, John Courtney, 109–10

natural law, 101, 181
Niebuhr, Reinhold, 15, 83
Nietzsche, Friedrich, 5–6, 114
Novak, Michael, 109

Oakeshott, Michael, 165, 177, 179

Paine, Tom, 84
Pascal, Blaise, 113
Pasternak, Boris
    resistance to fate, 22–23
Patterson, Orlando, 94

Paul, Saint, 20, 27, 31, 35, 89,
    92–95
Paul VI (pope), 119
personhood, 55–56, 65, 106–9,
    143–44, 157–58, 194
Pilate, Pontius, 245
Plato, 14, 38, 61,
    97, 100
postmodernism, 245
Protestant Reformation, 107, 120,
    123–24
    influence on modern democracy
        and human rights, 123, 129–34
    modern Protestant synthesis of
        Augustinian and Kantian
        ideas, 111
Pseudo-Dionysius, 100–101

Quakers, 107

Rawls, John, 8, 141, 166–67, 176, 179,
    193–206, 244
    and Kantian conception of
        equality, 8, 193, 203–5
    two basic principles of justice,
        197, 201
Rommen, Heinrich, 109
Rorty, Richard, 167
Rousseau, Jean-Jacques, 55

sanctity
    of persons, 143–45
Sartre, Jean-Paul, 239
Second Vatican Council, 106, 110,
    120, 228
Simmons, Menno, 106
Singer, Peter, 4–5, 7
    critique of, 147–49, 153–56
    and practical ethics movement, 4
    similarities with Ronald Dworkin,
        145–47

Socrates, 32, 34, 35, 39, 45
  "the true political art,"
     49–51
Stalin, Joseph, 15, 119

Taney, Chief Justice Roger, 158
Taylor, Charles, 208
teleology, 28
Tocqueville, Alexis de, 3,
     177–78, 184
totalitarianism, 3, 107, 215, 218
Twain, Mark, 184

Ulpian, 66
Universal Declaration of Human
     Rights, 109, 119, 131

Vinci, Leonardo da, 35
Voegelin, Eric, 83, 97, 103–5

Weil, Simone, 158–60
Wittgenstein, Ludwig, 186
Wright, Frank Lloyd, 38

Zwingli, Ulrich, 106